T0305701

Dose-Response Analysis Using R

Chapman & Hall/CRC
The R Series

For more information about this series, please visit: https://www.crcpress.com/go/the-r-series

Dose-Response Analysis Using R

Christian Ritz
Signe Marie Jensen
Daniel Gerhard
Jens Carl Streibig

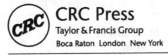

CRC Press
Taylor & Francis Group
Boca Raton London New York

CRC Press is an imprint of the
Taylor & Francis Group, an **informa** business

A CHAPMAN & HALL BOOK

CRC Press
Taylor & Francis Group
6000 Broken Sound Parkway NW, Suite 300
Boca Raton, FL 33487-2742

Library of Congress Cataloging-in-Publication Data

Names: Ritz, Christian, author.
Title: Dose-response analysis using R / by Christian Ritz, Signe M. Jensen,
Daniel Gerhard, Jens C. Streibig.
Description: Boca Raton, Florida : CRC Press, [2019] | Includes
bibliographical references and index.
Identifiers: LCCN 2019006744| ISBN 9781138034310 (hardback : alk.
paper) | ISBN 9781315270098 (e-book)
Subjects: LCSH: Drugs--Dose-response relationship. | Drugs--Testing--
Computer simulation.
Classification: LCC RM301.8 .R58 2019 | DDC 615.1--dc23
LC record available at https://lccn.loc.gov/2019006744

Visit the Taylor & Francis Web site at
http://www.taylorandfrancis.com

and the CRC Press Web site at
http://www.crcpress.com

Contents

Preface

The history of dose-response analysis goes back many hundred years. One of the more unusual applications is that numerous rulers had cupbearers who tried the ruler's food and drink to avoid poisoning and probably the demise of the regent. The dose-response was the survival/health of the cupbearer.

In more recent times, dose-response analysis was applied to data from controlled experiments where a limited number of doses of a toxic chemical compound were to be compared to a control group (dose 0) in terms of binary responses such as whether or not a treated insect was dead or alive after a certain time period (Finney, 1949). Later dose-response analysis crystallized into being a certain type of regression analysis. In the seminal work by Finney (1971) it is explained how to carry out the estimation in the so-called probit regression model through manual calculations. By the late 1970s dose-response analysis had been extended to log-logistic models for continuous response (Finney, 1979). In the beginning, such dose-response data were fitted through linearization (e.g., Streibig, 1981, 1983). Later nonlinear estimation of such models became available through add-ons and macros for spreadsheet programs (e.g., Vindimian *et al.*, 1983; Caux and Moore, 1997). General-purpose statistical software programs also included nonlinear estimation procedures but without any specific focus on dose-response analysis.

By 2005 the first version of the extension package *drc* was developed for the statistical programming environment **R** (R Core Team, 2018). Originally, it was developed for nonlinear fitting of log-logistic models that were routinely carried out in weed science (Ritz and Streibig, 2005). However, subsequently, the package has been modified and extended substantially, mostly in response to inquiries and questions from the user community. It has developed into a veritable ecosystem for dose-response analysis (Ritz *et al.*, 2015). Currently, such extensive functionality for dose-response analysis does not exist in any other statistical software. One of the problems that non-statistical scientists were facing in the past was that guestimates of nonlinear regression parameters had to be provided upfront before any estimation of parameters could take place; this was an insuperable problem for many practitioners. To a very large extent this problem has now been resolved in the package *drc* through the use of so-called self-starter routines.

The development of dose-response analysis has undergone dramatic changes from struggling with cumbersome more or less manual calculations and transformations with pen and paper to the blink-of-an-eye estimation of relevant parameters on any laptop.

A unified framework

The dose does not necessarily need to be a chemical compound. We define a dose (metameter) as any pre-specified amount of biological, chemical, or radiation stimuli or stress eliciting a certain, well-defined response. Other kinds of exposure or stress could also be imagined, e.g., time elapsed in germination experiments. However, in any case, the dose is a non-negative quantity.

Specifically, we define the response evoked by a specific dose as the quantification of a biologically relevant effect, and as such, it is subject to random variation. The most common type is a continuous response such as biomass, enzyme activity, or optical density. A binary or aggregated binary (binomial) response is also frequently used to describe results such as dead/alive, immobile/mobile, or present/absent (Van der Vliet and Ritz, 2013). The response may also be discrete as in a number of events observed in a specific time interval such as a number of juveniles, offspring, or roots (Ritz and Van der Vliet, 2009). We will have more examples in later chapters.

A key feature of dose-response analysis is that the experimenter or researcher has to have some a priori idea about the type of model function that would be relevant for the analysis of her/his dose-response data. In principle, many nonlinear model functions could be considered for describing how the average response changes over the range of doses considered. In practice, only a limited number of functions are used in the majority of applications. Specifically, we will focus on modeling average trends through mostly s-shaped or related biphasic functions. These functions reflect an *a priori* basic understanding of the causal relationship between the dose and the response, e.g., when a dose increases the response decreases between certain limits referred to as the lower and upper limits, respectively. S-shaped functions have turned out to be extremely versatile for describing various biological mechanisms; one key feature is that model parameters provide useful interpretations of observed effects within a biologically plausible framework. Specifically, dose-response analysis is often used for screening and ranking of compounds using estimated effective or lethal doses such as ED50 or LD50 (e.g., WHO, 2005).

The full specification of a statistical dose-response model involves both specifying the parametric model function and assumptions about the distribution of the responses, i.e., how they randomly fluctuate around the average value determined by an assumed model function. Distributional assumptions depend on the type of response observed. However, the same model functions may be meaningful for different types of responses, and this is the unifying feature of dose-response analysis: It involves dose-response models that are a collection of statistical models that have a certain mean structure in common. This is not a mathematical definition in any sense, but rather a definition driven by applications, which actually makes sense for a statistical methodology. Consequently, dose-response models encompass a range of statistical models that could be classified as nonlinear regression, generalized (non)linear regression, and parametric survival analysis. Perhaps this is one reason for dose-response analysis being neglected by many statisticians, as already pointed out many years ago (Finney, 1979).

What this book is and is not about

Nowadays the term dose-response is used in many different contexts. This book is about fitting and interpreting results obtained from fitting fully parametric nonlinear dose-response (regression) models. In short, this is how we define dose-response analysis and this book is meant to provide an introduction to this kind of dose-response analysis. We do not cover some areas of dose-response analysis that are still under development and where functionality is not yet available in **R**, such as dose-response analysis of data from mixture experiments and models for handling measurement error.

Some methods, which used to be part of a dose-response analysis, are intentionally not covered in the book: goodness-of-fit and lack-of-fit tests and other statistical tests that are used for assessing model assumptions. We prefer using statistical tests for evaluating research questions about differences.

This book neither covers analysis of variance of dose-response data nor estimation of linear trends, which are sometimes, and in some fields, referred to as dose-response analysis. In the past, and occasionally still, s-shaped dose-response trends or parts of them were approximated by means of linear regression models, e.g., parallel-line and slope-ratio assays, but such approaches are hardly needed anymore as was already pointed out a long time ago (Vølund, 1978). We also do not cover semi- or non-parametric approaches for modeling dose-response data. Finally, Bayesian methods for dose-response analysis are still in their infancy and not covered either.

How to read the book

The first five chapters deal with different types of dose-response data, and they may be read in arbitrary order as they are only loosely connected. However, there is a gradient such that more complex examples will be encountered in the later chapters. The last chapters are more specialized, covering recent advances, and therefore also more technical but still example-based. In examples, we will most often report estimates with corresponding standard errors in brackets, unless otherwise stated. We provide an appendix with more technical details and explanations for the interested reader, but most examples should be self-contained.

Above we praised the fact that modern dose-response analysis may be carried out in much the same way as linear regression analysis. This is indeed true, but as the estimation is intrinsically nonlinear, it can occasionally happen that the analysis is also less smooth and the user will need to provide more input. This is, in particular, the case when fitting more complex dose-response models. We provide some examples in Chapter 7.

Sometimes we analyze examples in the chapters in this book in several ways. This allows us to compare different approaches. In practice, a single approach should ideally be decided upon by the scientist's knowledge of the underlying biological mechanisms. We hope this book will be helpful in acquiring an informed opinion about when to use which approach.

Acknowledgment

We are fortunate in having some colleagues and experts, Florent Baty, Andrew Kniss, Andrea Onofri, Janine Wong, and Ming Yi, who kindly agreed to read sections or the entire manuscript. We are grateful for their valuable comments and correction of the substance and language. We would stress, however, that all these helpful people are in no way responsible for any mistakes which still occur; these are ours alone.

1

Continuous data

In this chapter, we show examples of how to analyze dose-response data that are continuous. It is a common type of dose-response data obtained in biology, toxicology, and many other fields. Specifically, a continuous response is a quantitative measurement that may take any value within a certain (possibly unlimited) range and is usually expressed in a quantitative unit such as colour, length, mass, and volume.

For continuous dose-response data, we will assume a statistical model where each response value y may be decomposed into two additive contributions. One contribution is determined or *predicted* by the corresponding dose through the assumed model function f, i.e., it will be the same contribution every time the same dose is applied; it is a fixed contribution for each dose. This contribution corresponds to the average response for a given dose. The other contribution is random, i.e., it will change from one replicate to the next, modifying the average response value in an unpredictable way. The randomness may, however, be characterized by a probability distribution that quantifies how likely the contribution is to take values in any given interval of response values. As these random contributions will modify the average response by adding or subtracting some value, we say that the probability distribution is centered around the mean (response). This statistical model may be written in the following way:

$$ y_i = f(x_i, \beta) + \varepsilon_i, \qquad i = 1, \ldots, n \tag{1.1} $$

with the fixed and random contributions adding up to the observed response value for each pair of dose and response (x_i, y_i), for a total of n measurements. It is common to assume that the random contributions, the ε_i's in Equation (1.1), follow a mean-zero normal distribution with an unknown residual standard deviation, which also is a model parameter to be estimated from the data. The residual standard error is a measure of the variation between measurements beyond what is explained by the assumed dose-response model function. We will also address how to deal with dose-response data that do not fully satisfy the above assumptions (see Subsection 1.1.3 and Subsection 1.1.4 for examples).

The model specification in Equation 1.1 relies on the assumption that the variation between replicates is the same for all doses (referred to as variance homogeneity). In this case, estimation may be carried out using nonlinear

1

least squares (see Section A.1 for more details) as the dose-response model is a special case of a nonlinear regression model (Ritz and Streibig, 2008).

In the examples below we will only specify the model function f and implicitly assume that a statistical model is defined through Equation (1.1). However, we will also address situations where the assumptions of normality and variance homogeneity are not fulfilled.

In this chapter, we use the following extension packages:

```
library(drc)
```

```
library(devtools)
install_github("DoseResponse/drcData")
library(drcData)
```

```
library(boot)
```

```
library(lmtest)
```

```
library(metafor)
```

```
library(sandwich)
```

1.1   Analysis of single dose-response curves

In the first example there are no replicates per dose, i.e., only a single response is obtained per dose. It can occur as a consequence of the experimental design, which may be a good thing if it means that more doses and fewer replicates were used. It can also happen because averages over the replicates were calculated per dose; this is a waste of data and should be avoided: All replicates should enter the analysis as shown in Subsection 1.1.2 and Subsection 1.1.3.

1.1.1   Inhibitory effect of secalonic acid

We want to carry out a dose-response analysis for the dataset `secalonic` shown below.

```
secalonic
```

```
##     dose rootl
## 1 0.000   5.5
## 2 0.010   5.7
```

```
## 3 0.019    5.4
## 4 0.038    4.6
## 5 0.075    3.3
## 6 0.150    0.7
## 7 0.300    0.4
```

Dose-response data were obtained from an experiment assessing the inhibitory effect of secalonic acid on plant growth (Gong *et al.*, 2004). The response values (in the variable named `rootl`) are root lengths in cm, and the dose values (`dose`) are in mM. Replicates were averaged per dose (as already pointed out above, this is in general not a good idea).

1.1.1.1 Fitting the model

In weed science a four-parameter log-logistic model is often used to describe dose-response relationships. We can use the model fitting function `drm()`, which is the pivotal function in the package *drc* for fitting dose-response models. Specifically, the response is specified on the left-hand side of the tilde ($\sim$) as the root length (`rootl`). The independent variable, which is denoted `dose`, is supplied to the right of the tilde. Next, we specify the dataset where the variables named `dose` and `rootl` are to be found using the argument `data`. The argument `fct = LL.4()` specifies a four-parameter log-logistic model where both lower and upper limits have to be estimated from the data. For continuous dose-response data it is not necessary to specify the argument `type` as the default is `type = "continuous"`. We store the resulting model fit in an object named `secalonic.LL.4`:

```
secalonic.LL.4 <- drm(rootl ~ dose,
                      data = secalonic,
                      fct = LL.4())
```

The first argument supplied to the function `drm()` is a *model formula* relating the response to the predictor. The second argument `data` is specifying the dataset where the variables `rootl` and `dose` are found. **R** will not automatically look for variables in the dataset `secalonic` because they are not in the *search path* and it is a good habit to specify the relevant dataset every time a model is fitted. The third argument `fct` specifies the dose-response model function that we want to fit. As there are 7 different doses, a four-parameter model may easily be fitted (usually as many doses as parameters are said to be required, but less will also do sometimes, possibly depending on the choice of model function and the number of replicates). The built-in function `LL.4()` in `drc` provides the four-parameter log-logistic model that is commonly used in toxicology (see Section B.1 for more details). In short, this model has four parameters: a lower limit, an upper limit, a parameter corresponding to ED50, and a parameter for the relative slope at the dose equal to ED50 (see Figure 1.1).

Note that upon execution of the above **R** lines, no output is produced. All information on the model fitted to the data is stored in the *object* named `secalonic.LL.4`, which is our choice for an informative name for the model fit; you are invited to use other names.

A plot of the observed response (`rootl` versus `dose`) and the corresponding fitted dose-response curve is obtained using the `plot` method.

Apart from the first argument (the model object `secalonic.LL.4`), the arguments in `plot` govern the layout of the plot. While the arguments `xlab`, `ylab` and `ylim` are self-explanatory (or see the help page `?par` for graphical parameters), the arguments `bp` and `broken` require a little more explanation. `broken` indicates the presence or absence of a break in the dose axis, in order to display that both 0 and the logarithm axis are shown and `bp` sets the value on the dose axis where the axis breaks. A break is needed in situations where zero concentrations/doses (x values) are combined with a logarithmic x-axis. The default value of `bp` is usually quite sensible, but in this particular

```
plot(secalonic.LL.4,
     bp = 1e-3, broken = TRUE,
     ylim = c(0, 7),
     xlab = "Dose (mM)",
     ylab = "Root length (cm)")
```

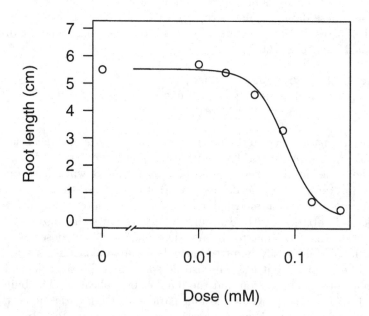

FIGURE 1.1
The four-parameter log-logistic model fitted to dose-response data from the dataset `secalonic` is plotted together with the original data (no replicates).

instance we must choose a smaller value to ensure that the bp value is smaller than all positive concentrations/doses (otherwise some observations are not displayed!). The argument `log = ""` may be used to switch off the default logarithmic dose axis.

A summary of the fit is obtained using the `summary` method when applied to the model fit `secalonic.LL.4`:

```
summary(secalonic.LL.4)

##
## Model fitted: Log-logistic (ED50 as parameter) (4 parms)
##
## Parameter estimates:
##
##                  Estimate Std. Error t-value  p-value
## b:(Intercept) 2.6542086  0.6962333  3.8122 0.0317398 *
## c:(Intercept) 0.0917852  0.3747246  0.2449 0.8223012
## d:(Intercept) 5.5297495  0.2010300 27.5071 0.0001055 ***
## e:(Intercept) 0.0803547  0.0078829 10.1935 0.0020121 **
## ---
## Signif. codes: 0 '***' 0.001 '**' 0.01 '*' 0.05 '.' 0.1 ' ' 1
##
## Residual standard error:
##
##   0.2957497 (3 degrees of freedom)
```

The output shows the type of model that was fitted and the parameter estimates for the four model parameters together with the corresponding (estimated) standard errors. Briefly, the parameter b, c, d, and e refer to the slope parameter for a dose equal to e, which is the dose resulting in a reduction halfway between the upper limit d and the lower limit c, which is also called ED50. We refer to Subsection B.1.1 for more details about the four-parameter log-logistic model.

For each parameter, there are also t-values, which are parameter estimates divided by their standard error, and the resulting p-values, looked up in an appropriate t distribution; each of them corresponds to testing the null hypothesis that the parameter is equal to 0 (not necessarily a relevant null hypothesis to consider). The estimated residual variance is also shown, although it is hardly reported in any publications, but it may still be useful for understanding variation in the experiment. Possibly, the most interesting parameter in the `summary` output is the parameter estimate for e; it is equal to 0.08 (0.0079).

We also see that the estimated lower limit, which is equal to 0.0918 with a standard error of 0.375, is not significantly different from zero (p-value $= 0.82$), possibly indicating that a three-parameter log-logistic model (with an assumed lower limit of 0) would also fit the data. However, such ad hoc data-driven model reduction is not meaningful and should be avoided. Assuming a lower limit equal to 0 should be based on *a priori* biological insights about the dose-response experiment, i.e., will root length ever be exactly 0 even for very high doses?

1.1.1.2   Estimation of arbitrary ED values

The function ED() calculates effective doses of your choice. Perhaps ED50 is not always a relevant parameter. For instance, in ecotoxicology a safe level for organisms may be defined using more protective levels such as ED10 or ED20. See Section A.10.1 for more about effective doses.

Any ED value is a function of the model parameters (for the four-parameter log-logistic model it is a function of the slope b and ED50), and it is possible to estimate any ED value and also the corresponding standard error from the model fit without having to re-parameterize and re-fit the model each time a new ED value has to be estimated. For instance, ED10 and ED20 based on the model fit secalonic.LL.4 are easily obtained using the following line:

```
ED(secalonic.LL.4, c(10, 20))
```

```
##
## Estimated effective doses
##
##           Estimate Std. Error
## e:1:10 0.0351149  0.0078689
## e:1:20 0.0476628  0.0074229
```

The output shows estimated ED values and corresponding (approximate) standard errors. A 10% reduction in the root length relative to the estimated upper and lower limits, which corresponds to a root length of 4.99, is achieved for a dose of 0.035 (0.0079) mM. One way of understanding the calculation is by reversing it using the function predict to predict the fitted value corresponding to the obtained dose:

```
predict(secalonic.LL.4,
        data.frame(dose = ED(secalonic.LL.4, c(10), display = FALSE)))
```

```
## Prediction
##   4.985953
```

The argument display = FALSE switches off showing the output from ED().

1.1.2   Data from a fish test in ecotoxicology

The OECD (2006, p. 65) guideline provides test data from a 21-day fish test using the test organism rainbow trout (*Oncorhynchus mykiss*). It is a standard toxicity experiment with 7 concentrations: 0 and 6 non-zero concentrations. The substance being tested at a range of concentrations is not known. There are 10 replicates per concentration. However, for some of the higher doses, several missing values occur so that the dataset contains only 61 observations (instead of 70). We note that ignoring such missing values may lead to a biased results, depending on the mechanism causing missingness. The measured response is the wet weight of the fish (in g). The dataset is available as the data frame O.mykiss.

Following OECD (2006, p. 80) we fit the two-parameter exponential decay model using the built-in function EXD.2(), which is a special case of the four-parameter log-logistic model. We use summary to obtain a summary of the model fit.

```
O.mykiss.EXD.2 <- drm(weight ~ conc,
                 data = O.mykiss,
                 fct = EXD.2(),
                 na.action = na.omit)

summary(O.mykiss.EXD.2)

##
## Model fitted: Exponential decay with lower limit at 0 (2 parms)
##
## Parameter estimates:
##
##                Estimate Std. Error t-value   p-value
## d:(Intercept)   2.846794   0.092526 30.7674 < 2.2e-16 ***
## e:(Intercept) 111.738614  33.196876  3.3659  0.001347 **
## ---
## Signif. codes: 0 '***' 0.001 '**' 0.01 '*' 0.05 '.' 0.1 ' ' 1
##
## Residual standard error:
##
##   0.5598508 (59 degrees of freedom)
```

Note that we specify the argument na.action to handle (in this case remove) the 9 missing values mentioned earlier. The resulting model fit plotted together with all data points (as indicated by the argument type = "all") is shown in Figure 1.2. Alternatively, the default argument type = "average" would imply plotting averages of replicates for each dose. Showing all data may be helpful in evaluating the model fit, whereas showing averages may be a better choice when reporting results.

The dataset is somewhat larger than in the previous example, so it makes some sense to investigate if the model assumptions are fulfilled. Graphical model checking can be based on the residual plot and QQ plot shown in Figure 1.3 and Figure 1.4, respectively. The visual assessment of the model fit

```
plot(O.mykiss.EXD.2,
     broken = TRUE,
     type = "all",
     xlim = c(0, 500), ylim = c(0, 4),
     xlab = "Concentration (mg/l)",
     ylab = "Weight (g)")
```

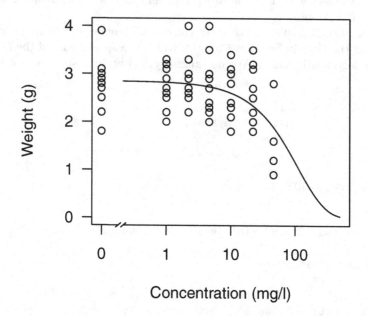

FIGURE 1.2
A two-parameter exponential decay model fitted to dose-response data from
a fish test (the dataset named O.mykiss) with up to 10 replicates per concentration (all replicates shown).

by the residual plot in Figure 1.3 indicates that the chosen model function
provides an appropriate description of the dose-response data because there is
random scatter above and below the reference line, which is the x axis, as the
residuals ought to be centered around 0. Furthermore, the residual plot shows
no indications of deviations from the model assumption of variance homogeneity as the scatter of points has the same spread across the entire range of the
x axis (which is similar to the range in the response values). Likewise, visual
assessment of the model fit by means of the QQ plot in Figure 1.4 indicates
that the normality assumption for the response values is appropriate because
the ranked (raw) residuals approximately match the corresponding expected
ordered values when assuming a normal distribution.

```
plot(fitted(O.mykiss.EXD.2),
     residuals(O.mykiss.EXD.2))

abline(h = 0, lty = 2)
```

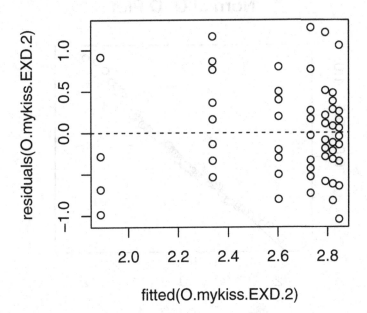

FIGURE 1.3
Residual plot for the two-parameter exponential decay model fitted to the dose-response data in the dataset O.mykiss. A reference line corresponding to the x axis has been added.

As for the previous example, the natural next step would be to estimate relevant ED values. However, we will not pursue this objective here.

1.1.3 Ferulic acid as an herbicide

As part of a larger experiment involving mixtures of several compounds, the effect of the natural compound ferulic acid as a potential herbicide on growth of perennial ryegrass was investigated (Inderjit *et al.*, 2002). The resulting dose-response data is found in the dataset ryegrass where the variable conc is the concentration of ferulic acid in mM and rootl is the resulting root length in cm. There are 7 concentrations, 6 replicates for concentration 0 and 3 replicates for all non-zero concentrations, in total 24 pairs of concentrations and response values. We start fitting a four-parameter log-logistic model to data as was also done in the original analysis reported by Inderjit *et al.* (2002).

```
qqnorm(residuals(O.mykiss.EXD.2))

abline(a = 0, b = sd(residuals(O.mykiss.EXD.2)))
```

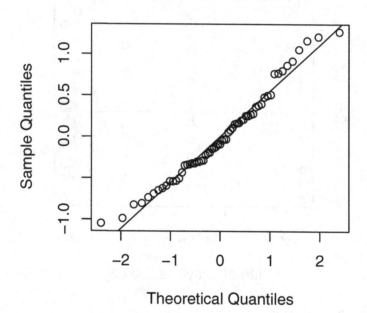

FIGURE 1.4
QQ plot for the two-parameter exponential decay model fitted to the dose-response data in the dataset O.mykiss. A reference line corresponding to the line with intercept 0 and slope equal to the empirical standard deviation of the residuals has been added.

```
ryegrass.LL.4 <- drm(rootl ~ conc,
                     data = ryegrass,
                     fct = LL.4())
```

The fitted dose-response curve together with the data is shown in Figure 1.5. We refer to Section C.1 for an example on how to make the plot by using the package *ggplot2* (Wickham, 2016).

Figure 1.5 shows that the variation in the response values is largest for mid-range concentrations, whereas the variation is less for smaller concentrations and much less for larger concentrations. Therefore, the model assumption about variance homogeneity may be questionable. We can explore this

```
plot(ryegrass.LL.4,
    broken = TRUE,
    type = "all",
    xlab = "Concentration (mM)",
    ylab = "Root length (cm)")
```

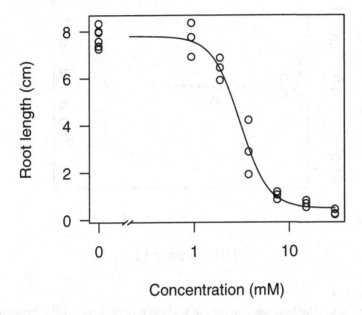

Concentration (mM)

FIGURE 1.5
Four-parameter log-logistic model fitted to the dataset ryegrass (all replicates shown).

observation further by means of graphical model checking: A residual plot (Figure 1.6) also shows a tendency towards increasing variation in the mid-range of response values (which corresponds to mid-range concentrations). The residual plot shows that the scatter is evenly distributed above and below the x axis, indicating that the chosen model function is adequately describing the average trend in the data. Therefore, we would not expect this slight model misspecification (variance heterogeneity) to have much effect on the estimated parameters, but it may affect the corresponding standard errors to a larger extent. It is worth pointing out that these departures from the model assumptions are unsurprising and may often be observed in a more or less pronounced way as a consequence of biological mechanisms (less variation under severe stress) and the experimental design (dilution series used for

Dose-response analysis using R

```
plot(fitted(ryegrass.LL.4), residuals(ryegrass.LL.4))

abline(h = 0, lty = 2)
```

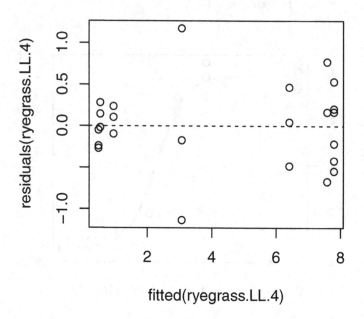

fitted(ryegrass.LL.4)

FIGURE 1.6
Residual plot for the four-parameter log-logistic model fitted to the ryegrass
dataset.

the concentrations). The QQ plot (not shown) does not reveal any departures
from normality.

One way to adjust for the model misspecification is to use robust standard
errors, which do not require that a modified model is fitted (see Section A.5).
It is a remedy applicable to the already fitted model. We can use the function
coeftest() from the extension package *lmtest* and rely on functionality from
the package *sandwich* to obtain robust standard errors.

```
coeftest(ryegrass.LL.4,
         vcov = sandwich)

##
## t test of coefficients:
##
##                 Estimate Std. Error t value  Pr(>|t|)
## b:(Intercept)    2.98222    0.47438  6.2865 3.882e-06 ***
## c:(Intercept)    0.48141    0.12779  3.7672  0.001212 **
```

```
## d:(Intercept)  7.79296    0.15311 50.8976 < 2.2e-16 ***
## e:(Intercept)  3.05795    0.26741 11.4355 3.170e-10 ***
## ---
## Signif. codes:  0 '***' 0.001 '**' 0.01 '*' 0.05 '.' 0.1 ' ' 1
```

To allow comparisons, the condensed summary output for the model fit (with naive standard errors) is shown below.

```
coef(summary(ryegrass.LL.4))
```

```
##                   Estimate Std. Error  t-value      p-value
## b:(Intercept) 2.9822191  0.4650623  6.412515 2.960347e-06
## c:(Intercept) 0.4814132  0.2121924  2.268758 3.450565e-02
## d:(Intercept) 7.7929583  0.1885672 41.327218 3.821922e-21
## e:(Intercept) 3.0579550  0.1857313 16.464401 4.267922e-13
```

The output shows a large decrease in the standard error for the parameter estimate of c (the lower limit) and an increase in the standard error for the estimated ED50. The standard errors for the estimates of b and d are less affected. Given Figure 1.5, the changes in the standard errors make sense: In the initial model fit where variance homogeneity was assumed, the increased variation observed in the mid-concentration range (where ED50 is found) was weighed down. The reduced variation observed for the larger concentrations mostly determining the lower limit (the parameter c) was weighed up, reflecting the assumption of variance homogeneity. The sandwich estimates do not underlie the assumption of variance homogeneity and, therefore, captures the actual variation in data to a higher degree. It is of course a balance. How much variation do we want to accommodate? Ideally only variation caused by some systematic effect or feature, not random variation.

The next example introduces yet another way to handle some types of model misspecification.

1.1.4   Glyphosate in barley

We consider (unpublished) data from an experiment where different doses of glyphosate (g a.i./ha) were applied to barley plants grown in a greenhouse. The endpoint was biomass (g/pot). We again fit a four-parameter log-logistic model to the data resulting in the fitted dose-response curve shown in Figure 1.7. The variation in biomass seems to decrease with increasing doses.

```
head(barley)
```

```
##       Dose weight
## 1  0.00000   57.2
## 2  0.00000   49.8
```

```
## 3 21.09375    62.2
## 4 21.09375    30.6
## 5 42.18750    40.9
## 6 42.18750    70.9

barley.LL.4 <- drm(weight ~ Dose,
                   data = barley,
                   fct = LL.4(),
                   na.action = na.omit)

summary(barley.LL.4)

##
## Model fitted: Log-logistic (ED50 as parameter) (4 parms)
##
## Parameter estimates:
##
##                 Estimate Std. Error t-value   p-value
## b:(Intercept)     9.7084    42.9166  0.2262   0.82430
## c:(Intercept)    11.1275     3.7803  2.9435   0.01068 *
## d:(Intercept)    52.0478     3.2487 16.0212 2.123e-10 ***
## e:(Intercept)   286.2600   209.6374  1.3655   0.19364
## ---
## Signif. codes:  0 '***' 0.001 '**' 0.01 '*' 0.05 '.' 0.1 ' ' 1
##
## Residual standard error:
##
##   9.241941 (14 degrees of freedom)
```

A residual plot also reveals the problem with the assumption of variance homogeneity: the variation in the response seems not to be constant (Figure 1.8). In some cases, a transformation could help to achieve variance homogeneity.

The logarithm transformation would be one option as it is often successful in removing the pattern observed in Figure 1.7: small variation in small predicted values and large variation in large predicted values. However, in order to preserve the assumed dose-response model, both the response and the predicted values based on the model have to be transformed. This technique was used for the logarithm transformation by Streibig (1983) and, in general terms, it is described as the transform-both-sides approach (Carroll and Ruppert, 1988, Chapter 4). It is also possible to search for the optimal transformation (within a family of transformations). We will consider Box-Cox transformations, which are power functions with negative and positive exponents (but also including the logarithm); see Section A.3 for more details. It should be mentioned that there is some evidence that the transform-both-sides approach may lead to inappropriate fitted dose-response curves in some

```
plot(barley.LL.4,
     broken = TRUE,
     type = "all",
     xlab = "Dose (g a.i./ha)",
     ylab = "Biomass (g/pot)")
```

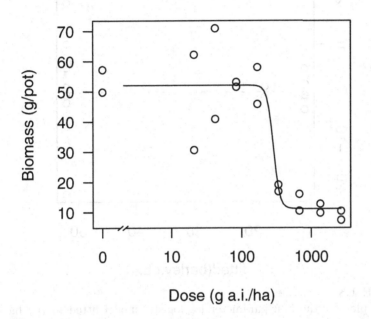

FIGURE 1.7
The four-parameter log-logistic model fitted to the barley data (`barley`).

cases (Ritz and Van der Vliet, 2009): so it is not an approach that we would like to recommend for general use.

We can obtain the model fit for the optimal so-called Box-Cox transformation by refitting the model using the function `boxcox()`. The argument `method` specifies that we want to estimate and apply the optimal power exponent, which is determined from the slightly more general one-way ANOVA model rather than directly from the dose-response model (as there is a computational gain in doing so).

```
barley.LL.4.bc <- boxcox(barley.LL.4,
                         method = "anova",
                         plotit = FALSE)
```

```
summary(barley.LL.4.bc)
```

```
plot(fitted(barley.LL.4), residuals(barley.LL.4))

abline(h = 0, lty = 2)
```

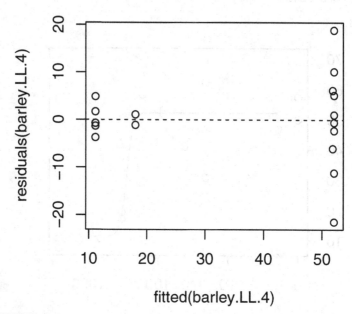

FIGURE 1.8
Residual plot for the four-parameter log-logistic model fitted to the barley data (`barley`).

```
##
## Model fitted: Log-logistic (ED50 as parameter) (4 parms)
##
## Parameter estimates:
##
##                 Estimate Std. Error t-value    p-value
## b:(Intercept)     4.6567     4.3207  1.0778   0.299362
## c:(Intercept)    10.5303     1.1542  9.1231 2.875e-07 ***
## d:(Intercept)    51.4583     5.4983  9.3590 2.109e-07 ***
## e:(Intercept)   250.8884    52.3177  4.7955  0.000285 ***
## ---
## Signif. codes:  0 '***' 0.001 '**' 0.01 '*' 0.05 '.' 0.1 ' ' 1
##
## Residual standard error:
##
```

```
##   0.1121892 (14 degrees of freedom)
##
## Non-normality/heterogeneity adjustment through Box-Cox
##      transformation
##
## Estimated lambda: -0.25
## Confidence interval for lambda: [-0.576, 0.370]
```

The optimal power exponent (λ) for the Box-Cox transformation is -0.25, which is significantly different from 1 (no transformation) as the corresponding confidence interval does not include 1. However, the value 0 (corresponding to the log-transformation) is included in the confidence interval. Except for the slope parameter b, none of the parameter estimates changed dramatically due to the transformation.

Alternatively, we may also directly specify the appropriate power exponent using the argument bcVal in the model specification. This approach of making an informed choice is to be preferred over estimating the optimal transformation as we did above. Perhaps only a few transformations are really relevant in practice, e.g., the logarithm transformation and, occasionally, the square root transformation. The drawback of this approach might be that some a priori information about the distribution of the response is required (possibly from other similar experiments).

```
barley.LL.4.log <- drm(weight ~ Dose,
                       data = barley,
                       fct = LL.4(),
                       na.action = na.omit,
                       bcVal = 0)


summary(barley.LL.4.log)

##
## Model fitted: Log-logistic (ED50 as parameter) (4 parms)
##
## Parameter estimates:
##
##                  Estimate Std. Error t-value   p-value
## b:(Intercept)     6.6523     8.8818   0.7490  0.466271
## c:(Intercept)    10.7738     1.1385   9.4628 1.843e-07 ***
## d:(Intercept)    51.1127     4.4105  11.5890 1.461e-08 ***
## e:(Intercept)   269.2678    76.8634   3.5032  0.003513 **
## ---
## Signif. codes:  0 '***' 0.001 '**' 0.01 '*' 0.05 '.' 0.1 ' ' 1
##
## Residual standard error:
```

```
##
##   0.2457367 (14 degrees of freedom)
##
## Non-normality/heterogeneity adjustment through Box-Cox
##        transformation
##
## Specified lambda: 0
```

We can add the fitted dose-response curve obtained using the transform-both-sides approach with the logarithm transformation in the plot of the fitted dose-response curve using untransformed data. The two fitted curves agree quite well (see Figure 1.9).

```
plot(barley.LL.4.log,
     add = TRUE,
     lty = 2)
```

Finally, we may choose to stay with our initial model but using sandwich estimates for the standard errors as in the example above. It should, however, be noticed that the sandwich standard errors rely on the mean structure, i.e.,

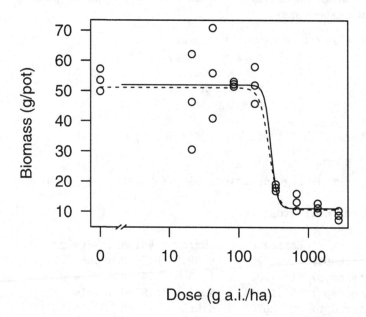

FIGURE 1.9
The four-parameter log-logistic model fitted to the barley data (`barley`), both untransformed data (solid line) and when using a transform-both-sides approach with the logarithm transformation (dashed line).

the model function, being correctly specified, which may be hard to judge for the present data example with sparse information in the middle of the curve.

```
coeftest(barley.LL.4,
         vcov. = sandwich)

##
## t test of coefficients:
##
##                 Estimate Std. Error t value   Pr(>|t|)
## b:(Intercept)    9.7084    33.8435   0.2869     0.7784
## c:(Intercept)   11.1275     1.1026  10.0918 8.341e-08 ***
## d:(Intercept)   52.0478     4.0530  12.8417 3.899e-09 ***
## e:(Intercept)  286.2600   165.3541   1.7312     0.1054
## ---
## Signif. codes:  0 '***' 0.001 '**' 0.01 '*' 0.05 '.' 0.1 ' ' 1
```

In summary both the transform-both-sides approach and the use of robust standard errors lead to sensible changes in the standard errors of the parameter estimates for the lower and upper limits. The standard error became smaller for the lower limit and it became larger for the upper limit as compared to the standard errors from the initial model barley.LL.4, which assumed variance homogeneity. For the slope and ED50 parameter estimates, all approaches lead to smaller standard errors, but they are still mostly large compared to the magnitude of the corresponding estimate, indicating that there is essentially no information in the data to determine the slope and EC50 parameters. At best, only EDxx for large percentages xx may be reliably estimated and such quantities are usually not that relevant.

1.1.5 Lower limits for dose-response data

For growth-related measurements, the response sometimes does not approach a lower limit of 0 even though larger and larger doses are applied. One explanation is that an organism being exposed to a toxic compound at a certain time during its development has already had a growth before exposure and this growth may or may not be preserved for a longer time depending on the mode of action of the toxic compound. Another explanation could be drug resistance. Consequently, the lower limit of the corresponding dose-response curve may be positive, reflecting growth before exposure. The two following examples will illustrate the concept. However, there may also be other reasons for the absence or presence of a lower limit such as a systematic measurement error that prevents observation of response values asymptotically approaching 0. In any case, such *a priori* information about one aspect of the dose-response relationship should ideally be incorporated when choosing the model function. Below we consider two illustrative examples.

The first example uses data from an experiment where ryegrass plants were treated with a mixture of commercial herbicides that prevents further growth but leaves the plants green and viable for a long time. The herbicides are acetolactate synthase inhibitors that do not block photosynthesis *per se*, but prevent the photosynthetic production from making the plant grow. The biomass of the plants was measured on the day of spraying (where the mixture would have no visible effect) and 15 days after spraying (for a range of doses). The data, which are unpublished, are found in the dataset ryegrass2.

```
head(ryegrass2)
```

```
##   dose biomass day
## 1    0    77.5   0
## 2    0    78.0   0
## 3    0    75.0   0
## 4    0   214.4  15
## 5    0   215.4  15
## 6    0   227.5  15
```

We fit a four-parameter log-logistic model to the subset of data containing information on the measurements 15 days after spraying.

```
ryegrass2.LL.4 <- drm(biomass ~ dose,
                      data = subset(ryegrass2, day == "15"),
                      fct = LL.4())
```

Figure 1.10 shows the fitted dose-response curve with a horizontal line added showing the mean biomass level before spraying (at day 0).

In this instance, the biomass production (growth) at the time of spraying (day 0) closely corresponds to the lower limit due to the mode of action of the herbicide.

The second example involves the contact herbicide diquat, which was applied to red fescue, and after 16 days the biomass was measured (unpublished data). The herbicide is a desiccant that kills the plant instantaneously. It means the degradation of the plant commences immediately after the spraying. Therefore, for high doses, we would expect biomass to approach 0.

```
head(red.fescue, 4)
```

```
##   dose day biomass
## 1    0   0    45.0
## 2    0   0    69.0
## 3    0  16   137.0
## 4    0  16   102.0
```

```
plot(ryegrass2.LL.4,
     broken = TRUE,
     ylim = c(0, 250),
     xlab = "Dose (g a.i./ha)",
     ylab = "Weed biomass (g/pot)")

abline(h = mean(subset(ryegrass2, day == "0")[["biomass"]]),
       lty = 2)
```

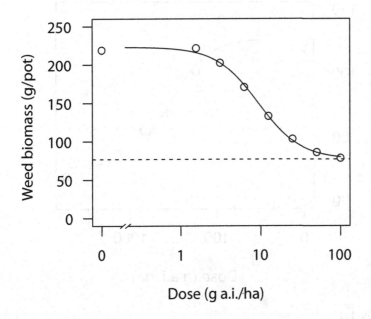

FIGURE 1.10
Fitted four-parameter log-logistic model for biomass of ryegrass 15 days after being sprayed with a mixture of herbicides that stop growth but leave affected plants green (using the dataset `ryegrass2`). The dashed line indicates biomass on day 0, the day when the experiment was sprayed with the herbicide mixture.

We fit a four-parameter log-logistic model.

```
red.fescue.LL.4 <- drm(biomass ~ dose,
                       data = subset(red.fescue, day == "16"),
                       fct = LL.4())
```

```
plot(red.fescue.LL.4,
     broken = TRUE,
     ylim = c(0, 150),
     xlab = "Dose (g a.i./ha)",
     ylab = "Biomass (g/pot)")

abline(h = mean(subset(red.fescue, day =="0")[["biomass"]]),
       lty = 2)
abline(h = coef(red.fescue.LL.4)["c:(Intercept)"], lty = 3)
```

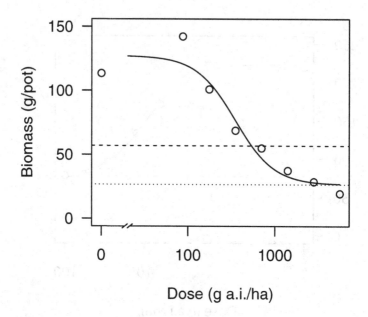

FIGURE 1.11
Fitted four-parameter log-logistic model for biomass of red fescue 16 days after being sprayed with the desiccant herbicide diquat that kills the plant quickly. Dashed broken line indicates the biomass level at the time of spraying (day 0) and the dotted line shows the estimated lower limit after 16 days.

Figure 1.11 shows the fitted dose-response curve together with a horizontal line representing the level of biomass at the time of spraying (day 0), which does not coincide with the estimated lower limit that the mean response is approaching for large doses. In this case, it reflects a different mode of action of the herbicide. It is worth noting that the data still seem to indicate that there is a positive lower limit, but it is not reflecting growth before exposure.

1.1.6   A hormesis effect on lettuce growth

Hormesis is a stimulatory response to low levels of stress, such as low concentrations of organic or inorganic chemicals or radiation. Hormesis has been observed for various organisms such as animals, humans, microbiota, and plants; see Cedergreen *et al.* (2005) and Beckon *et al.* (2008) for more details.

We re-analyze data from an experiment where lettuce plants were grown in nutrient solutions containing different concentrations of dissolved isobutylalcohol (mg/L) (van Ewijk and Hoekstra, 1993). Shoot weight (g) was measured after 21 days. Seven concentrations (including the control) were used. For each concentration duplicate measurements were obtained. The data are found in the dataset `lettuce`. The entire dataset is shown below.

`lettuce`

```
##       conc weight
## 1     0.00  1.126
## 2     0.00  0.833
## 3     0.32  1.096
## 4     0.32  1.106
## 5     1.00  1.163
## 6     1.00  1.336
## 7     3.20  0.985
## 8     3.20  0.754
## 9    10.00  0.716
## 10   10.00  0.683
## 11   32.00  0.560
## 12   32.00  0.488
## 13  100.00  0.375
## 14  100.00  0.344
```

The variables `conc` and `weight` contain the concentration and corresponding weight measurements. A scatterplot of the data is shown in Figure 1.12. A warning is issued because of the argument `log = "x"`, which imposes a logarithmic concentration axis that allows us to better appreciate the hormesis effect: there is a fairly clear inverse j-shape with an increase at low concentrations before showing the expected decreasing trend for higher concentrations.

We fit the four-parameter Brain-Cousens hormesis model with the lower limit fixed at 0 as we assume that there will not be any growth for high concentrations. The special feature of this hormesis model, as well as other hormesis models, is the additional model parameter that quantifies the degree of hormesis. For the Brain-Cousens model, this parameter is denoted f, and the interpretation is that $f = 0$ implies no hormesis effect, whereas $f > 0$ implies some degree of hormesis, the larger the value the larger the effect. However, the actual value of f cannot directly be understood by the scale of the response. The parameters b and d have the same interpretation as for the

```
plot(weight ~ conc,
    data = lettuce, log = "x",
    xlab = "Isobutylalcohol concentration (mg/L)",
    ylab = "Weight (g)")
```

```
## Warning in xy.coords(x, y, xlabel, ylabel, log): 2 x values
<= 0 omitted from logarithmic plot
```

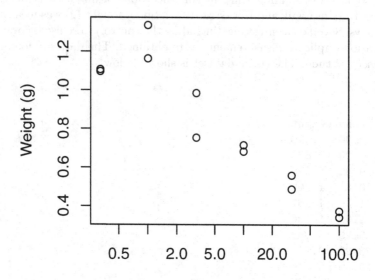

FIGURE 1.12
Data in the `lettuce` dataset showing a hormesis effect.

log-logistic models: b is proportional to the slope at the concentration equal to e, which, however, is not equal to EC50, and d is the upper asymptote or limit of the dose-response curve (see Equation B.12 in Subsection B.1.2 for more details). This model was also used in the original analysis by van Ewijk and Hoekstra (1993). The built-in model function BC.4() invokes this model.

```
lettuce.BC.4 <- drm(weight~conc,
                    data = lettuce,
                    fct = BC.4())
```

Figure 1.13 shows the original data with the fitted dose-response curve superimposed. The model appears to fit the data well.

The summary output shows that the hormesis parameter f is not significantly different from 0 (p-value is 0.129), which means that we cannot reject the hypothesis of no hormetic effect using the dataset `lettuce`.

```
plot(lettuce.BC.4,
     broken = TRUE,
     xlab = "Isobutylalcohol concentration (mg/L)",
     ylab = "Weight (g)")
```

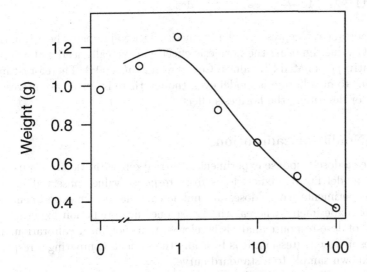

FIGURE 1.13
The fitted concentration-response curve for the four-parameter Brain-Cousens model fitted to the dataset lettuce, shown together with the data (average per concentration).

```
summary(lettuce.BC.4)

##
## Model fitted: Brain-Cousens (hormesis) with lower limit fixed
##       at 0 (4 parms)
##
## Parameter estimates:
##
##                 Estimate Std. Error t-value    p-value
## b:(Intercept)   1.282812   0.049346 25.9964  1.632e-10 ***
## d:(Intercept)   0.967302   0.077123 12.5423  1.926e-07 ***
## e:(Intercept)   0.847633   0.436093  1.9437    0.08059 .
## f:(Intercept)   1.620703   0.979711  1.6543    0.12908
```

```
## ---
## Signif. codes: 0 '***' 0.001 '**' 0.01 '*' 0.05 '.' 0.1 ' ' 1
##
## Residual standard error:
##
##   0.1117922 (10 degrees of freedom)
```

More importantly, the presence of a hormesis effect will impact the estimation of any EC value. Ignoring the hormesis effect will typically lead to too small (conservative) estimated EC values (Cedergreen *et al.*, 2005). Therefore it may be relevant to fit a hormesis model even though there is *per se* no interest in assessing or describing the hormesis effect.

1.1.7   Nonlinear calibration

Sometimes a dose-response experiment is carried out with the aim to use the resulting model fit to predict doses from response values observed in subsequent experiments where doses are unknown. The former experiment is a calibration experiment, whereas the latter ones are prediction experiments. This kind of dose-response analysis is referred to as nonlinear calibration, and it involves inverse regression. It is basically the same as comparing a response of an unknown sample to a standard curve.

We revisit the following data example first considered by Racine-Poon (1988): To explore degradation of an agrochemical in soil samples it was applied in 0-10 cm depth in 7 different doses, including dose 0 (g/ha). The observed response is the weight (mg) of a nasturtium plant after 3 weeks. This calibration experiment was repeated 6 times (so an improved analysis would model variation between the 6 runs explicitly).

The first 12 lines of the dataset look like this:

```
head(nasturtium, 12)
```

```
##       conc rep  wt
## 1    0.000   1 920
## 2    0.025   1 919
## 3    0.075   1 870
## 4    0.250   1 880
## 5    0.750   1 693
## 6    2.000   1 429
## 7    4.000   1 200
## 8    0.000   2 889
## 9    0.025   2 878
## 10   0.075   2 825
## 11   0.250   2 834
## 12   0.750   2 690
```

As in the original analysis, we fit a three-parameter log-logistic model:

```
nasturtium.LL.3 <- drm(wt ~ conc, data = nasturtium, fct = LL.3())

summary(nasturtium.LL.3)


##
## Model fitted: Log-logistic (ED50 as parameter) with lower
##      limit at 0 (3 parms)
##
## Parameter estimates:
##
##                Estimate Std. Error t-value    p-value
## b:(Intercept)   1.350256   0.113557  11.891 1.518e-14 ***
## d:(Intercept) 897.862776  13.844884  64.852 < 2.2e-16 ***
## e:(Intercept)   1.576200   0.095694  16.471 < 2.2e-16 ***
## ---
## Signif. codes: 0 '***' 0.001 '**' 0.01 '*' 0.05 '.' 0.1 ' ' 1
##
## Residual standard error:
##
##  55.55935 (39 degrees of freedom)
```

Backfitting is a quick way to see how good the calibration model is. We use the function `backfit()` in *drc* that takes the model fit object as the only argument.

```
backfit(nasturtium.LL.3)

## Warning in log(exp(-tempVal/parmVec[5]) - 1): NaNs produced

##        dose  Estimate
## [1,] 0.000       NaN
## [2,] 0.025 0.1152911
## [3,] 0.075 0.1522799
## [4,] 0.250 0.2418827
## [5,] 0.750 0.7209820
## [6,] 2.000 2.0729493
## [7,] 4.000 3.8933864
```

The agreement is good, although for low doses (large response values) estimated doses are too large. The warning message may be ignored as it simply means it is not possible to estimate dose 0.

Let us assume that a prediction experiment resulted in response values 690, 693, and 722; this is similar to but not identical to what Racine-Poon (1988)

did. For each single response value, we can use the function ED() for estimating
the corresponding dose with a 95% confidence interval. For instance, for the
value 690 we get:

```
ED(nasturtium.LL.3, 690, type = "absolute", interval = "delta")

##
## Estimated effective doses
##
##          Estimate Std. Error    Lower     Upper
## e:1:690 0.648194   0.070708 0.505174 0.791214
```

Note that the argument type = "absolute" is essential. By default, the argument is type = "relative", which is suitable for estimating effective doses.
The 95% confidence interval of the estimated dose is $[0.505, 0.791]$. However,
this interval is likely somewhat too narrow as it does not incorporate the variation in the response value. Likewise, we could also estimate the dose based
on the mean of the response values:

```
ED(nasturtium.LL.3, (690+693+722)/3, type = "absolute",
   interval = "delta")

##
## Estimated effective doses
##
##                        Estimate Std. Error    Lower     Upper
## e:1:701.666666666667 0.613385   0.069337 0.473137 0.753633
```

One way to incorporate variation in the response values, but also utilize that
three values were recorded, is through a bootstrap approach where estimated
doses are repeatedly computed for randomly sampled values from a normal
distribution assumed for the mean of the three response values. Specifically,
we will assume that the mean of 690, 693, and 722 follow a normal distribution
with mean $(690 + 693 + 722)/3$ and standard deviation $56/\sqrt{3}$ where 56 is the
residual standard error from the above model fit.

To do a bootstrap, we use the extension package *boot*. As a first attempt
we will do a crude parametric bootstrap, which will incorporate the variation
in the response values, but it will not propagate the uncertainty on parameter
estimates when doing inverse regression. The key function boot() is specified
as follows: The first argument is the data, i.e., the mean response. The second
argument is the R function that converts the data value into an estimated
concentration; this is essentially ED() but being wrapped up in a function environment to allow only one value to vary. The third argument is the function
that returns randomly sampled values from the assumed normal distribution
of the mean; it is relying on the R function rnorm(). The fourth argument is

needed when giving the third argument. The last argument specifies the number of times to randomly draw mean values (it is common to use 1000). The function `set.seed()` is used to ensure that the bootstrap procedure results in the same results every time (based on the same pseudo-random numbers).

```
set.seed(201806061)
nasturtium.boot.res1 <- boot((693+722+690)/3,
                             statistic = function(simyVal){
                               ED(nasturtium.LL.3,
                                  simyVal,
                                  type = "absolute",
                                  display = FALSE)[1]
                             },
                             ran.gen = function(yVal, mle){
                               rnorm(1, yVal, 55.55935/sqrt(3))
                             },
                             sim = "parametric",
                             R = 1000)

summary(nasturtium.boot.res1)

##       R original  bootBias   bootSE bootMed
## 1 1000   0.61338 0.0028725 0.098303 0.61955
```

A 95% percentile bootstrap confidence interval may be obtained using the function `boot.ci()`, also from the package *boot*. Specifically, we will use the basic bootstrap confidence interval, which includes the middle 95% of the estimated dose values based on generated response values, i.e., the middle 950 values among the 1000 being generated by the function `boot()` (Davison and Hinkley, 1997).

```
boot.ci(nasturtium.boot.res1, type = "basic")

## BOOTSTRAP CONFIDENCE INTERVAL CALCULATIONS
## Based on 1000 bootstrap replicates
##
## CALL :
## boot.ci(boot.out = nasturtium.boot.res1, type = "basic")
##
## Intervals :
## Level       Basic
## 95%   ( 0.4200,  0.8032 )
## Calculations and Intervals on Original Scale
```

The resulting 95% confidence interval becomes $[0.42, 0.8]$, which is somewhat wider than the one we found by simply using `ED()`, $[0.47, 0.75]$.

An improved parametric bootstrap approach would not only generate values for the mean response in the prediction model but also for all response values used in the calibration model, as such an approach would ensure that a 95% confidence interval of the dose of interest is based on all the variation present in the analysis. For each generated set of $42 + 3 = 45$ response values, the three-parameter log-logistic model should be fitted and the estimated concentration obtained from inverse regression; this is what is happening below in the second argument, based on randomly generated response values.

```
set.seed(201806062)
nasturtium.boot.res2 <- boot(c(nasturtium[["wt"]], 690, 693, 722),
                      statistic = function(yValues){
                          ED(drm(head(yValues, -3) ~ conc,
                                 data = nasturtium,
                                 fct = LL.3()),
                             mean(tail(yValues, 3)),
                             type = "absolute",
                             display = FALSE)[1]
                      },
                      ran.gen = function(yVal, mle){
                          rnorm(42+3,
                                c(fitted(nasturtium.LL.3),
                                  690, 693, 722), 55.55935)
                      },
                      sim = "parametric",
                      R = 1000)

boot.ci(nasturtium.boot.res2, type = "basic")

## BOOTSTRAP CONFIDENCE INTERVAL CALCULATIONS
## Based on 1000 bootstrap replicates
##
## CALL :
## boot.ci(boot.out = nasturtium.boot.res2, type = "basic")
##
## Intervals :
## Level      Basic
## 95%   ( 0.3780,  0.8184 )
## Calculations and Intervals on Original Scale
```

The resulting 95% bootstrap confidence interval is slightly wider than the previous one, implying that not much additional variation is picked up by repeating all the steps of the nonlinear calibration. The above results are similar to the ones derived by Racine-Poon (1988) through a completely different approach.

1.2   Analysis of multiple dose-response curves

In this section, we consider two data examples with two treatment groups.
In both examples below, the main interest lies in comparing treatments in
terms of some feature of the dose-response curves that may be captured by
model parameters or a derived parameter. It is common to compare ED50
values between treatments, either in terms of differences or ratios depending
on which quantification is most relevant, e.g., in toxicology and weed science
it is often the ratio that is of interest.

   In the first example, there is only a single dose-response sub-experiment
for each of two treatments, implying that there is no way to separate random
variation between dose-response curves (due to various unobserved differences
in the execution of each dose-response sub-experiment) from systematic differences between treatments. Consequently, only weak claims on treatment
differences may be made based on such an experimental design. In the second
example, there are two replicated dose-response sub-experiments for each of
two treatments, allowing a stronger claim about a possible treatment difference. In a later chapter (Chapter 7) we will show how to analyze dose-response
data for more complex, possibly multiway factorial, experimental designs.

1.2.1   Effect of an herbicide mixture on *Galium aparine*

Small plants of cleavers (*Galium aparine*), growing in pots (one plant per pot)
in a large greenhouse, were sprayed with the herbicide phenmedipham either
alone or in a mixture with methyl oleate. For both herbicide treatments the
same 11 doses (g/ha) were used. There were 10 replicates per dose and per
treatment except for dose 0 where there were 40 replicates. Dose 0 was shared
between the two treatments, but in the dataset (`G.aparine`) the controls were
assigned to one of the treatments (it does not matter which one as long as the
dose-response model assumes a shared control). The plants were allowed to
grow in the greenhouse for 14 days after treatment, and then the dry matter
(weight in mg/pot) was measured. The experiment is described in more detail
by Cabanne *et al.* (1999). The first 6 lines of the dataset are shown below.

```
head(G.aparine)
```

```
##   dose drymatter treatment
## 1    0      1146         1
## 2    0      1005         1
## 3    0       756         1
## 4    0      1108         1
## 5    0       956         1
## 6    0       989         1
```

The variable `drymatter` contains the measured dry weight per pot, the variable `dose` contains doses of the two herbicide treatments, and the variable `treatment` encodes the two herbicide treatments: 1 corresponds to phenmedipham alone and 2 corresponds to the mixture of phenmedipham and methyl oleate; the latter is an adjuvant that does not have any effect in the plants.

For each of the two herbicide treatments, a single dose-response sub-experiment with replicates per dose was carried out. Such an experimental design implies that the herbicide treatment effects and the sub-experiment effects (if present) are confounded; had there been multiple dose-response sub-experiments per herbicide treatment these two effects could have been disentangled.

We fit a joint model based on the entire dataset including both herbicide treatments. Actually, as there is a shared control group, there is no other option than a joint model to avoid that the control group counts twice in the analysis. Again, we use the model fitting function `drm()`, including the additional argument named `curveid` that provides information on the grouping in the data and also including the argument `pmodels` that for each of the four model parameters b, c, d, and e (in that order) specifies if the grouping should be applied (~`treatment`) or no grouping should be used, i.e., a single common model parameter shared by all groups (~1). As there is a shared control group we have to insist on a shared parameter d for the upper limit. The model specification looks like this.

```
G.aparine.LL.4 <- drm(drymatter ~ dose,
                  curveid = treatment,
                  data = G.aparine,
                  fct = LL.4(),
                  pmodels = list(~treatment,
                               ~treatment,
                               ~1,
                               ~treatment))
```

So for each model parameter, we use a model formula specification similar to what is used for `lm()` in **R**. These model formulas are combined in a list; alternatively a data frame could be supplied. This means that we can compare the two herbicide treatments in terms of any of the model parameters b, c, or e. However, in practice, only comparisons of ED50 values (the parameters e in this example) are of interest.

Figure 1.14 shows the fitted dose-response curves together with average data per dose. The model seems to describe the dose-response relationships quite well. A residual plot and QQ plot could be used for a more detailed evaluation of the model assumptions in the same way as seen for a single dose-response curve in Subsection 1.1.2.

```
plot(G.aparine.LL.4,
     broken = TRUE,
     xlab = "Dose (g/ha)",
     ylab = "Dry weight (mg/pot)")
```

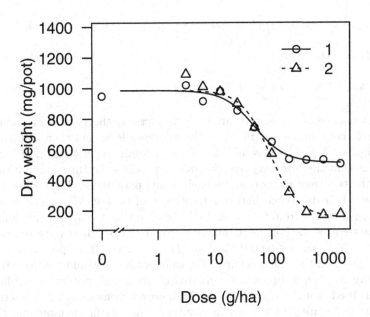

FIGURE 1.14
The fitted dose-response curves for the four-parameter log-logistic model (with
a shared control group) fitted to the dataset G.aparine. Average data per
concentration are also shown.

As we assume a four-parameter log-logistic model per herbicide treatment,
but with the constraint that the upper limit parameter is shared, we estimate
a total of 7 model parameters (shown in the summary output below).

```
summary(G.aparine.LL.4)

##
## Model fitted: Log-logistic (ED50 as parameter) (4 parms)
##
## Parameter estimates:
##
##                Estimate Std. Error  t-value    p-value
## b:(Intercept)   1.61291    0.33330   4.8392 2.373e-06 ***
## b:treatment2    0.13809    0.37301   0.3702 0.7115667
```

```
## c:(Intercept)    509.50242    23.25903   21.9056 < 2.2e-16 ***
## c:treatment2    -357.58391    34.71802  -10.2997 < 2.2e-16 ***
## d:(Intercept)    984.88794    12.63336   77.9593 < 2.2e-16 ***
## e:(Intercept)     50.80033     7.87857    6.4479 6.468e-10 ***
## e:treatment2      42.64599    10.94359    3.8969 0.0001274 ***
## ---
## Signif. codes:  0 '***' 0.001 '**' 0.01 '*' 0.05 '.' 0.1 ' ' 1
##
## Residual standard error:
##
##    111.403 (233 degrees of freedom)
```

As a consequence of the specification ~ **treatment**, the treatment coming first in alphabetic order was taken as the reference level and then compared to the other level, just as it would happen for a similar specification in lm(). This means that the summary output directly provides the three comparisons between the two treatments (one for each model parameter). For the parameter b there is a difference between treatment of 0.14 (0.37), which is not significantly different from 0 ($p = 0.71$), indicating that the slopes are similar for the two treatments. For the parameters c and e (ED50) there are significant differences: -358 (35; $p < 0.0001$) and 43 (11; $p = 0.00013$), respectively.

Thus, based on the difference in ED50 values only, we would conclude that the mixture of phenmedipham and methyl oleate is less potent than phenmedipham used alone. This conclusion is, however, somewhat contradicting the picture in Figure 1.14 where it is clear that the mixture is more effective as it reduces dry matter much more than phenmedipham alone, which does not kill the plant completely even at the highest doses. The explanation is that the comparison of ED50 values is relative to the estimated lower and upper limits, and in this example the lower limits are quite different. So to get the full picture, the lower limits also need to be considered (and perhaps even the slopes). Simply relying on ED50 values (or any other EDxx values) may be misleading. However, the interpretation also becomes more difficult as differences in several model parameters have to be taken into consideration.

Occasionally interest lies in comparing the entire dose-response curve between treatments in one go, corresponding to looking at all three of the above-mentioned comparisons. The approximate F-test offers a combined statistical test for such a global comparison. It requires fitting a reduced model where a single dose-response curve was fitted based on the pooled data from the two herbicide treatments.

```
G.aparine.LL.4.pooled <- drm(drymatter ~ dose,
                       data = G.aparine,
                       fct = LL.4())
```

The F-test may now be invoked using the **anova()** method.

```
anova(G.aparine.LL.4.pooled, G.aparine.LL.4)
```

```
##
## 1st model
## fct:      LL.4()
## pmodels: 1 (for all parameters)
## 2nd model
## fct:      LL.4()
## pmodels: ~treatment, ~treatment, ~1, ~treatment
## ANOVA table
##
##             ModelDf      RSS Df F value p value
## 1st model      236  4927249
## 2nd model      233  2891677  3  54.673   0.000
```

As reported above, two out of three comparisons between the two treatments of the individual model parameters gave significant results. Therefore, it is not surprising that the global test is also significant ($p < 0.0001$): the p-value from the global test may be thought of as a kind of weighted average of these individual p-values.

1.2.2   Glyphosate and bentazone treatment of *Sinapis alba*

The potency of the two herbicides glyphosate and bentazone in white mustard (*Sinapis alba*) was compared in an experiment reported by Christensen *et al.* (2003). There were two independent sub-experiments for each herbicide with the same seven doses plus an untreated control except for one glyphosate sub-experiment where an eighth dose was included (also with four replicates).

The experimental layout was planned as a completely randomized design with four replicates for each herbicide dose except for the untreated control (dose 0) where 8 replicates were used. Unlike the previous example in Subsection 1.2.1 the herbicide effects and the sub-experiment effects are not confounded.

Data are provided in the dataset *S.alba.comp*.

```
head(S.alba.comp)
```

```
##   exp herbicide dose drymatter  Tf  area  Fo   Fm
## 1 ben1 bentazone    0       4.1 200 31200 278 1662
## 2 ben1 bentazone    0       3.4 230 30600 278 1670
## 3 ben1 bentazone    0       2.6 210 27400 299 1646
## 4 ben1 bentazone    0       3.5 260 34600 288 1715
## 5 ben1 bentazone    0       4.3 200 31000 272 1651
## 6 ben1 bentazone    0       4.2 240 31400 286 1681
```

The first four columns are: `exp` denotes the sub-experiment (four levels), `herbicide` denotes the herbicide applied, `dose` is the dose of the herbicide applied (g a.i./ha), and `drymatter` is the response (in g/pot). There are four more columns in the dataset, but they will not be used here.

We fit a joint model based on data from all four sub-experiments. Ideally, we would fit a dose-response mixed-effects model that would treat the sub-experiment variation as a separate source of variation. However, only having two sub-experiments per herbicide treatment is not much and it may be difficult to fit such a mixed model. We will come back to mixed models in Chapter 7. Instead, we will look at two simpler approaches.

We may consider a joint model where we ignore the information about the sub-experiments or, put in another way, pooling data from the two sub-experiments for each herbicide. This approach corresponds to assuming that the double number of replicates were used per dose (which is of course not true). A joint model is convenient if we want to compare the two herbicides. There is, however, no compelling reason for having a joint model encompassing data from all sub-experiments. Moreover, it has been shown that, in theory, estimated model parameters will be the same for a joint model and for separate models per herbicide (Fang and Zhang, 2014). In practice, numerical issues may lead to slight differences. Therefore, as an alternative, we may consider separate models per sub-experiment and seek to combine them.

1.2.2.1   A joint dose-response model

We fit a joint model using `drm()`, but including the additional argument `curveid` that provides information on the treatment groups in the data. For each group a four-parameter log-logistic model may describe the average dose-response relationship. It implies that a total of $4 \cdot 2 = 8$ parameters have to be estimated.

```
S.alba.LL.4 <- drm(drymatter ~ dose,
               curveid = herbicide,
               data = S.alba.comp,
               fct = LL.4())
```

If there had been *a priori* knowledge available about some of the model parameters being the same for both herbicides, then the argument `pmodels` could have been used to incorporate such assumptions: Perhaps the lower and upper limits for the two herbicides are identical, whereas slopes and ED50 parameters are different from herbicide to herbicide? It depends on what we know about the experiment before collecting data.

The summary output shows that the lower and upper limits for the herbicides are fairly similar, indicating that it may be meaningful to compare the herbicides in terms of ED50 levels.

```
summary(S.alba.LL.4)
```

```
##
## Model fitted: Log-logistic (ED50 as parameter) (4 parms)
##
## Parameter estimates:
##
##                 Estimate Std. Error t-value   p-value
## b:bentazone     4.421705   1.376978  3.2112  0.001658 **
## b:glyphosate    1.606429   0.322669  4.9786 1.949e-06 ***
## c:bentazone     0.679894   0.092323  7.3643 1.673e-11 ***
## c:glyphosate    0.894469   0.138322  6.4666 1.756e-09 ***
## d:bentazone     4.018895   0.107033 37.5481 < 2.2e-16 ***
## d:glyphosate    3.874354   0.122103 31.7302 < 2.2e-16 ***
## e:bentazone    21.293475   1.348860 15.7863 < 2.2e-16 ***
## e:glyphosate   46.245932   6.379062  7.2496 3.074e-11 ***
## ---
## Signif. codes:  0 '***' 0.001 '**' 0.01 '*' 0.05 '.' 0.1 ' ' 1
##
## Residual standard error:
##
##   0.4952302 (133 degrees of freedom)
```

Figure 1.15 shows the fitted dose-response curves together with averages per herbicide and dose. The model fit seems to be more or less appropriate.

The estimated relative potency based on the ED50s for the two herbicides is obtained using the function EDcomp(), which takes the model fit as the first argument and the ED levels (provided as percentages) to be compared as the second argument. Additionally, we specify the argument interval = "delta" to obtain confidence intervals based on the delta method.

```
EDcomp(S.alba.LL.4, c(50, 50), interval = "delta")
```

```
##
## Estimated ratios of effect doses
##
##                              Estimate    Lower    Upper
## bentazone/glyphosate:50/50    0.46044  0.32220  0.59868
```

Bentazone is approximately twice as potent as glyphosate. If the argument interval = "delta" would be left out, then the p-value for testing the ratio equal to 1 would be shown (it is very small).

We can also compare the two herbicides in terms of the difference in ED50 values using the function compParm(), which provides comparisons as differences or ratios. Here the difference is estimated by specifying "-" as the third

```
plot(S.alba.LL.4,
     broken = TRUE,
     xlab = "Dose (g a.i./ha)",
     ylab = "Dry matter (g/pot)")
```

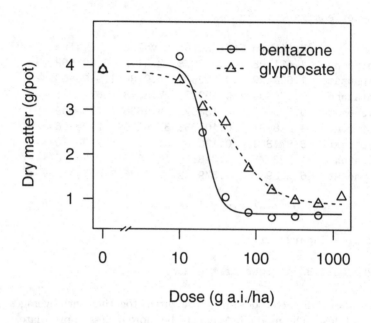

FIGURE 1.15
Four-parameter log-logistic model fitted to data on the effect of glyphosate
and bentazone on growth of white mustard (bentazone: solid line and open
circles, glyphosate: dashed line and triangles).

argument. The first two arguments are the model fit and the parameter of
interest.

```
compParm(S.alba.LL.4, "e", "-")

##
## Comparison of parameter 'e'
##
##                       Estimate Std. Error t-value    p-value
## bentazone-glyphosate  -24.9525  6.5201     -3.827   0.0001988 ***
## ---
## Signif. codes:  0 '***' 0.001 '**' 0.01 '*' 0.05 '.' 0.1 ' ' 1
```

Bentazone has a significantly smaller ED50 as compared to glyphosate, but
also a significantly steeper slope as shown below using compParm().

```
compParm(S.alba.LL.4, "b", "-")

##
## Comparison of parameter 'b'
##
##                       Estimate Std. Error t-value p-value
## bentazone-glyphosate    2.8153     1.4143  1.9906 0.04857 *
## ---
## Signif. codes: 0 '***' 0.001 '**' 0.01 '*' 0.05 '.' 0.1 ' ' 1
```

Note that comparison of the same two parameters by means of a difference
and a ratio (such as the above two ED50 values) will usually not result in
the same p-value even though the same null hypothesis is being tested. The
reason is the use of the delta method to obtain the estimated standard error
for the ratio: a nonlinear change of scale of the parameter estimates will lead
to approximate standard errors (see also Section A.10).

1.2.2.2 Fitting separate dose-response models

The two-step approach proposed by Jiang and Kopp-Schneider (2014) is an
alternative to nonlinear mixed-effects models for dose-response analysis.

The first step consists of fitting a separate dose-response model for data
from each of the four independent sub-experiments. In principle the models
fitted to data from each independent sub-experiment need not be the same
as long as the same parameter of interest may be estimated from all models.
From each model fit, estimates of parameters of interest (with corresponding estimated standard errors) are combined into a new dataset along with
information about treatments.

In a second step, these estimates are used as response values in a meta-
analytic random effects model where the experimental design is accounted
for through the use of fixed and random effects. In contrast to a usual linear
mixed model, the residual standard error is not estimated in the meta-analytic
random effects model. Instead, it is assumed to be non-constant and equal
to the estimated standard errors corresponding to the estimates. Inferential
procedures such as pairwise comparisons based on approximate Wald-type
U-tests are available, just like for an ordinary linear mixed model.

```
S.alba.LL.4.b1 <- drm(drymatter ~ dose,
                data = subset(S.alba.comp, exp == "ben1"),
                fct = LL.4())

S.alba.LL.4.b2 <- drm(drymatter ~ dose,
                data = subset(S.alba.comp, exp == "ben2"),
                fct = LL.4())
```

```
S.alba.LL.4.g1 <- drm(drymatter ~ dose,
                      data = subset(S.alba.comp, exp == "gly1"),
                      fct = LL.4())

S.alba.LL.4.g2 <- drm(drymatter ~ dose,
                      data = subset(S.alba.comp, exp == "gly2"),
                      fct = LL.4())
```

The next step is to extract the estimated ED50 values with the corresponding standard errors for each sub-experiment: We define a 4×2 matrix of NAs. Then we fill in row by row the estimated ED50 and the corresponding standard errors (coef() and summary() and square brackets to extract the values in row 4 and columns 1 and 2).

```
ed50.estimates <- matrix(NA, 4, 2)

ed50.estimates[1, ] <- coef(summary(S.alba.LL.4.b1))[4, 1:2]
ed50.estimates[2, ] <- coef(summary(S.alba.LL.4.b2))[4, 1:2]
ed50.estimates[3, ] <- coef(summary(S.alba.LL.4.g1))[4, 1:2]
ed50.estimates[4, ] <- coef(summary(S.alba.LL.4.g2))[4, 1:2]

ed50.estimates
```

```
##           [,1]     [,2]
## [1,] 29.26479 2.065501
## [2,] 18.85085 3.967966
## [3,] 25.56620 5.793800
## [4,] 62.73827 6.390966
```

Finally, we convert the matrix to a data frame with specified column names (est and se) and a column with information about the treatments: the first two rows contain estimates for the sub-experiments for bentazone and the last two rows for glyphosate.

```
ed50.estimates <- as.data.frame(ed50.estimates)
names(ed50.estimates) <- c("est", "se")
ed50.estimates <- cbind(ed50.estimates,
                        treatment = c("bentazone", "bentazone",
                                      "glyphosate", "glyphosate"))

ed50.estimates
```

```
##         est       se treatment
## 1 29.26479 2.065501  bentazone
## 2 18.85085 3.967966  bentazone
```

```
## 3 25.56620 5.793800 glyphosate
## 4 62.73827 6.390966 glyphosate
```

The estimates may be pooled into combined estimates using functionality from the **R** package *metafor* (Viechtbauer, 2010). Specifically we use the function `rma()`, which takes the estimated ED50 values as the first argument and the corresponding *squared* standard errors as the second argument; the smaller the standard error, the more weight will be assigned to the corresponding estimate. The treatment variable is specified by means of a formula (as also for many other model fitting functions) using the argument `mods`. Finally, the argument `data` is used for providing the dataset where the variables given in the first three arguments are found.

Specifically, we fit a weighted version of a one-way analysis of variance model for ED50 (`est`) with squared standard errors of estimated ED50 values as weights (`se`), using the argument `mods = ~ treatment`. These variables are found in the dataset `ed50estimates`, which we defined above.

```
S.alba.ED50 <- rma(est, se^2, mods = ~ treatment,
                   data = ed50.estimates)
```

A condensed version of the summary output shows the estimated difference in ED50 between the two herbicides: the estimated ED50 is 19.8 (18.7) larger for glyphosate than for bentazone. This difference is not significant ($p = 0.29$).

```
round(coef(summary(S.alba.ED50)), 3)
```

```
##                    estimate     se  zval  pval    ci.lb  ci.ub
## intrcpt              24.147 12.945 1.865 0.062   -1.224 49.518
## treatmentglyphosate  19.819 18.675 1.061 0.289  -16.784 56.421
```

Results from the joint and separate models disagree somewhat. The estimated differences in ED50 are fairly similar. However, incorporating variation between sub-experiments, which is the more appropriate approach, makes it more difficult to claim a significant difference as more variation in the data is captured by this dose-response analysis.

2

Binary and binomial dose-response data

In this chapter, we enter the classical area of dose-response analysis, which owes much to the seminal work by Finney (1971) as well as later contributions by Morgan (1992) among others.

A binomial response is a sum of independent binary responses: 0/1, no/yes, or absent/present; a binary response is a special case of a binomial response (see also Subsection A.2.1). The total number of binary responses per concentration or dose is decided upon as part of the experimental design and, hence, it is known in advance, prior to observing the responses. These total numbers need not be the same for all concentrations.

In some cases, the dose-response models for binomial data will be special cases of generalized linear models for binomial data (e.g., experiments eliciting the full range from 0% to 100% response). However, in other cases the dose-response models may be seen as extensions corresponding to generalized linear models with link functions depending on one or more parameters (e.g., experiments where the control group will not show a 0% or 100% response). Moreover, dose-response analysis of binomial data is based on statistical models that describe the mean trend on the probability scale, not on the log odds scale as would typically be the case for a generalized linear model for binomial data, e.g., logistic regression (McCullagh and Nelder, 1989, Chapter 4).

It is not unusual that the assumption of independence is not satisfied. For instance, several organisms could share a container or several plants or seeds could be placed in the same pot. Such departures may manifest themselves through so-called under- or, more commonly, over-dispersion where the variation in the dose-response data is not adequately described by a model relying on the assumption of independence. Consequently, the routine analysis will need to be modified, either by attempting to augment the dose-response model to allow extra-dispersion or, indirectly, by modifying standard errors into robust ones but otherwise not changing the dose-response model. Which approach to choose may to some extent depend on the data. Graphical model checking by means of residuals is not very useful for binomial data and, thus, model checking is more difficult. We will rely on visual assessment of plots of fitted dose-response curves together with observed proportions.

In this chapter, we use the following extension packages:

```
library(drc)
```

```
library(devtools)
```

```
install_github("DoseResponse/drcData")
library(drcData)

library(multcomp)
```

2.1 Analysis of single dose-response curves

2.1.1 Acute inhalation toxicity test

Racine *et al.* (1986) analyze data from a routine acute inhalation toxicity test
where 20 animals were exposed to 4 doses (mg/ml of an unknown substance),
5 animals per dose. The entire dataset is shown below.

```
acute.inh

##   dose total num.dead
## 1  422     5        0
## 2  744     5        1
## 3  948     5        3
## 4 2069     5        5
```

We fit a two-parameter log-logistic model using the model fitting function
drm(). The proportions of dead animals (num.dead/total), which is the response, are specified on the left-hand side of the tilde ($\sim$). The independent
variable, which is denoted dose, is specified on the right-hand side of the
tilde. As we specify the response as proportions, we also need to give the
totals (total) through the argument weights. It informs the estimation procedure about the relative weighting of the binomial response values according
to the number of underlying binary responses (in case the response is binary
the weights would all be equal to 1 and they would not need to be specified). Next, we specify the dataset with the variables named num.dead, total,
and dose. The argument fct = LL.2() specifies a two-parameter log-logistic
model where the lower limit is fixed at 0 and the upper limit is fixed at 1.
Finally, the argument type indicates the type of response data to be analyzed.
This is different as compared to continuous dose-response data where it was
not necessary to specify this argument as the default is type = "continuous".
We store the resulting model fit in an object named acute.inh.LL.2:

```
acute.inh.LL.2 <- drm(num.dead/total ~ dose,
                      weights = total,
                      data = acute.inh,
                      fct = LL.2(),
                      type = "binomial")
```

```
plot(acute.inh.LL.2, broken = TRUE,
     xlim = c(0, 10000), ylim = c(0, 1),
     ylab = "Proportion dead",
     xlab = "Dose (mg/ml)")
```

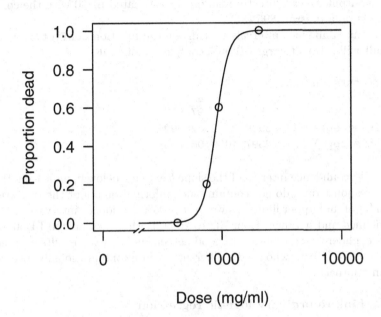

FIGURE 2.1
Two-parameter log-logistic model fitted to the dataset `acute.inh`.

A plot of the original data and the fitted dose-response curve can give a visual impression of how well the model fits the data, and with such a small dataset it is possibly the only reasonable means of assessing the model. The plot is shown in Figure 2.1. The model seems to provide a good fit to the data.
    To see the parameter estimates we use the **summary** method.

```
summary(acute.inh.LL.2)
```

```
##
## Model fitted: Log-logistic (ED50 as parameter) with lower
##     limit at 0 and upper limit at 1 (2 parms)
##
## Parameter estimates:
##
##                 Estimate Std. Error t-value p-value
## b:(Intercept)   -7.9301     5.0812 -1.5607  0.1186
```

```
## e:(Intercept) 895.2982    83.5547 10.7151  <2e-16 ***
## ---
## Signif. codes: 0 '***' 0.001 '**' 0.01 '*' 0.05 '.' 0.1 ' ' 1
```

From the output we can directly read off the estimated LD50 with the corresponding standard error: 895 (84).

To obtain confidence intervals we can use the function `confint()`, which by default will return (marginal) 95% confidence intervals.

```
confint(acute.inh.LL.2)
```

```
##                      2.5 %       97.5 %
## b:(Intercept) -17.88909     2.028992
## e:(Intercept) 731.53397  1059.062485
```

The 95% confidence interval of the slope b extends below 0, indicating that the dose-response data do not contain much information about the transition between lower and upper limits. However, the 95% confidence interval of LD50 is well defined and it ranges from 732 to 1059. Both the estimated LD50 and the 95% confidence intervals are in good agreement with the results obtained by Racine *et al.* (1986), who used a different or more computationally involved Bayesian approach.

2.1.1.1   Link to ordinary logistic regression

To see the link to ordinary logistic regression, we can fit exactly the same model by means of the function `glm()`:

```
acute.inh.glm <- glm(cbind(num.dead, total-num.dead) ~ log(dose),
                     data = subset(acute.inh, dose > 0),
                     family = binomial)
```

The resulting **summary** output looks like this:

```
coef(summary(acute.inh.glm))
```

```
##             Estimate Std. Error   z value   Pr(>|z|)
## (Intercept) -53.90152   34.34623 -1.569358 0.1165646
## log(dose)     7.93001    5.08122  1.560651 0.1186062
```

As the parameterization used in `glm()` differs from the one used in `drm()`, the parameter estimates will not all be the same: The estimated intercept in the logistic regression model fit is equal to $b \cdot \log(e)$ ((`-7.9301` * `log(895.2982)` = `-53.90213`). The estimated slope of `log(dose)` is identical to the estimated slope parameter b in the above two-parameter log-logistic model fit except for the change in sign. It is exactly the same model fit except for small numerical differences due to different estimation procedures being used. For a related example using logistic regression, we refer to Venables and Ripley (2002, pp. 190–194).

2.1.2 Tumor incidence

Shao (2012) analyzes binomial dose-response data describing liver tumor incidence in female Sprague-Dawley rats that were exposed to the chemical 2,3,7,8-tetrachlorodibenzo-p-dioxin (TCDD). There are 6 non-zero concentrations of TCDD and approximately 50 rats were exposed to each concentration. The entire dataset is shown below.

```
liver.tumor
```

```
##    conc total incidence
## 1  0.00    49         0
## 2  2.56    48         0
## 3  5.69    46         0
## 4  9.79    50         0
## 5 16.57    49         1
## 6 29.70    53        13
```

Fitting a two-parameter log-logistic model to the dataset `liver.tumor` may be carried out using the following lines.

```
liver.tumor.LL.2 <- drm(incidence/total ~ conc,
                 weights = total,
                 data = liver.tumor,
                 fct = LL.2(),
                 type = "binomial")
```

The resulting **summary** output shows the estimated slope and EC50, where EC50 may be interpreted as the concentration of TCDD resulting in a total incidence of 50%:

```
summary(liver.tumor.LL.2)
```

```
##
## Model fitted: Log-logistic (ED50 as parameter) with lower
##      limit at 0 and upper limit at 1 (2 parms)
##
## Parameter estimates:
##
##               Estimate Std. Error t-value   p-value
## b:(Intercept)  -4.9750     1.6897 -2.9443  0.003237 **
```

```
## e:(Intercept)    37.1774      4.1838  8.8859 < 2.2e-16 ***
## ---
## Signif. codes: 0 '***' 0.001 '**' 0.01 '*' 0.05 '.' 0.1 ' ' 1
```

It may be much more relevant to estimate EC5 or EC10 to get quantities that reflect realistic levels of exposure. Such EC values are so-called derived parameters, which are functions of the model parameters, and they can be estimated using the function ED().

```
ED(liver.tumor.LL.2, c(5, 10), interval = "delta")
```

```
##
## Estimated effective doses
##
##           Estimate Std. Error   Lower   Upper
## e:1:5      20.5705     2.5294 15.6129 25.5281
## e:1:10     23.9041     1.9778 20.0278 27.7804
```

The argument `interval` specifies the method applied for calculating confidence intervals. Here we ask for intervals based on the delta method (Piegorsch and Bailer, 2005, pp. 436–437), which are commonly reported, even though they are approximate, only reaching exactly 95% coverage for large sample sizes.

It is important to realize that by choosing the two-parameter log-logistic model, the lower and upper asymptotes are *a priori* fixed at the values 0 and 1, respectively. It means that any response obtained for dose 0 is redundant and will not be used in the estimation at all. For the same reason, large doses will also only contribute little to the model fit. In other words, the choice of model already contributes information about the dose-response relationship and this piece of information cannot be updated based on the data as there is no relevant parameter in LL.2() that could utilize such information (the lower limit is fixed at 0). One way to see that dose 0 data add nothing to the analysis is to repeat the analysis without dose 0:

```
liver.tumor.LL.2.no.zero <- drm(incidence/total ~ conc,
                                weights = total,
                                data = subset(liver.tumor, conc > 0),
                                fct = LL.2(),
                                type = "binomial")
```

Estimates and standard errors are exactly the same as for the model fitted to the entire dataset:

```
summary(liver.tumor.LL.2.no.zero)
```

```
##
## Model fitted: Log-logistic (ED50 as parameter) with lower
##       limit at 0 and upper limit at 1 (2 parms)
##
```

```
## Parameter estimates:
##
##                  Estimate Std. Error t-value    p-value
## b:(Intercept)     -4.9750     1.6897 -2.9443   0.003237 **
## e:(Intercept)     37.1774     4.1838  8.8859 < 2.2e-16 ***
## ---
## Signif. codes: 0 '***' 0.001 '**' 0.01 '*' 0.05 '.' 0.1 ' ' 1
```

In contrast, removal of one or more of the non-zero concentrations where the incidence is 0 will change the results (although not that much) as observations for these concentrations are used for estimating the parameters *b* and *e*. We revisit this data example in Subsection 6.1.3.

2.1.3   Earthworm toxicity test: Abbott's formula

This subsection provides an example of dose-response analysis in case the data exhibits natural mortality in the control group (dose 0). If there is any biological or other reasons to expect natural mortality then it should be reflected in the choice of dose-response model.

In contrast to the previous examples, the dose-response data in the present example require an analysis that goes beyond the standard logistic regression model. Because, by design of the experiment, the lower limit of the dose-response curve cannot be assumed to be equal to 0 (the built-in assumption for any standard logistic regression model). In the past, re-scaling of the response, which is referred to as applying Abbott's correction or formula, has been a convenient, but an inappropriate way to deal with natural mortality (e.g., Environment Canada, 2005, p. 46). It is convenient because it reduces the subsequent analysis to fitting a (standard) two-parameter dose-response model, like the ones fitted in the previous subsections. It is inappropriate because it introduces downwards or upwards bias (Hoekstra, 1987). Any such pre-processing of data prior to fitting a dose-response model should be avoided; this was already pointed out by Finney (1971, Chapter 7). Instead, a dose-response model with a non-zero lower limit should be fitted.

Hoekstra (1987) analyze data from an earthworm toxicity test with 6 concentrations of the herbicide chloroacetamide. For each concentration, 40 earthworms were exposed to the herbicide and subsequently the number of dead earthworms was counted. The control or natural mortality was $3/40 = 7.5\%$.

chlorac

```
##   conc total num.dead
## 1    0    40        3
## 2   10    40        5
## 3   20    40        6
```

```
## 4    40     40         38
## 5    80     40         40
## 6   160     40         40
```

In order to incorporate natural mortality, we use a three-parameter dose-response model where there is an additional model parameter describing the proportion of natural mortality. Following Hoekstra (1987) we fit a three-parameter log-normal model including a parameter for the lower limit (corresponding to the natural mortality), but fixing the upper limit at 1 as was also the case for the two-parameter models in the previous examples. This is an example of a generalized nonlinear model: a logistic regression model with a parameter-dependent extension of the usual probit link function (Finney, 1971). The corresponding built-in function in *drc* is named LN.3u(), which is short for LN.4(fixed = c(NA, NA, 1, NA)).

```
chlorac.LN.3u <- drm(num.dead/total ~ conc,
                     weights = total,
                     data = chlorac,
                     fct = LN.3u(),
                     type = "binomial")
```

The fitted dose-response curve captures the dose-response trend in the data adequately, as shown in Figure 2.2.

Below, the summary output and the 95% confidence intervals are shown.

```
summary(chlorac.LN.3u)

##
## Model fitted: Log-normal with upper limit at 1 (3 parms)
##
## Parameter estimates:
##
##                  Estimate Std. Error t-value   p-value
## b:(Intercept)    4.603773   1.043813  4.4105 1.031e-05 ***
## c:(Intercept)    0.099988   0.033573  2.9783  0.002899 **
## e:(Intercept)   28.291922   2.271962 12.4526 < 2.2e-16 ***
## ---
## Signif. codes: 0 '***' 0.001 '**' 0.01 '*' 0.05 '.' 0.1 ' ' 1

confint(chlorac.LN.3u)

##                     2.5 %      97.5 %
## b:(Intercept)   2.55793762   6.6496084
## c:(Intercept)   0.03418668   0.1657886
## e:(Intercept)  23.83895875  32.7448861
```

```
plot(chlorac.LN.3u, broken = TRUE,
     xlim = c(0, 1000), ylim = c(0, 1),
     ylab = "Proportion dead",
     xlab = "Concentration (mg/kg)")

abline(a = coef(chlorac.LN.3u)[2], b = 0, lty = 2)
```

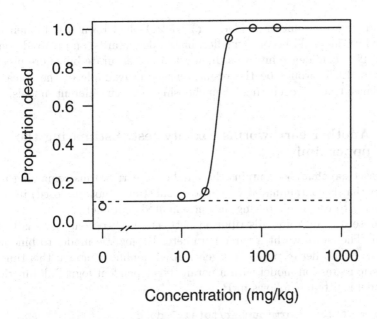

FIGURE 2.2
Two-parameter log-logistic model fitted to the dataset `chlorac`. The dashed line shows the estimated non-zero lower limit.

The estimated natural mortality, which is the parameter estimate for c converted and rounded to an integer percentage, is equal to 10% with a 95% confidence interval ranging from 3.4% to 17%. The estimated EC50 is equal to 28.29 with a 95% confidence interval ranging from 24 to 33; Hoekstra (1987) found a very similar result.

The EC50 corresponds to a 50% increase between the estimated lower limit and the fixed upper limit of 1, that is the concentration resulting in 50% mortality beyond the natural mortality. It does not correspond to the concentration resulting in a total mortality of 50%, which is an EC value that is defined in absolute terms based on the probability scale and not relative to limits partly or fully estimated from the data. For binomial data these absolute EC values are often more relevant than the relative ones and they may also be estimated using the function `ED()`.

```
ED(chlorac.LN.3u, 50 /100, type = "absolute")
```

```
##
## Estimated effective doses
##
##          Estimate Std. Error
## e:1:0.5   27.4464     2.3155
```

If instead a two-parameter model (e.g., LN.2()) had been fitted, then the estimated EC50 would become smaller, biased downwards, and it would have narrower 95% confidence intervals. In short, a less accurate but more precise estimate of EC50 would be the result; this is an example of the so-called bias-variance tradeoff occurring when choosing between different models.

2.1.4 Another earthworms toxicity test: Estimating the upper limit

The dataset earthworms contains the number of earthworms remaining in a container that is contaminated with a toxic substance (not disclosed) instead of migrating to the neighbouring uncontaminated container.

For dose 0, a fifty-fifty distribution between the two containers is to be expected. Therefore, we fit a three-parameter log-logistic model to binomial data. This is another example of a generalized nonlinear model; this time it is a logistic regression model with a parameter-dependent logit link function. This model is fitted as follows in **R**.

```
earthworms.LL.3 <- drm(number/total ~ dose,
                    weights = total,
                    data = earthworms,
                    fct = LL.3(),
                    type = "binomial")
```

```
summary(earthworms.LL.3)
```

```
##
## Model fitted: Log-logistic (ED50 as parameter) with lower
##     limit at 0 (3 parms)
##
## Parameter estimates:
##
##                 Estimate Std. Error t-value   p-value
## b:(Intercept) 1.505679   0.338992   4.4416 8.928e-06 ***
## d:(Intercept) 0.604929   0.085800   7.0505 1.783e-12 ***
## e:(Intercept) 0.292428   0.083895   3.4856  0.000491 ***
## ---
## Signif. codes: 0 '***' 0.001 '**' 0.01 '*' 0.05 '.' 0.1 ' ' 1
```

Perhaps even better (truer to the experimental design) would be to fit a log-logistic model where the upper limit is not estimated but instead fixed at the value 0.5. This is achieved using the following **R** lines:

```
earthworms.LL.3.fixed <- drm(number/total ~ dose,
                        weights = total,
                        data = earthworms,
                        fct = LL.3(fixed = c(NA, 0.5, NA)),
                        type = "binomial")

summary(earthworms.LL.3.fixed)
```

```
##
## Model fitted: Log-logistic (ED50 as parameter) with lower
##      limit at 0 (2 parms)
##
## Parameter estimates:
##
##                Estimate Std. Error t-value    p-value
## b:(Intercept) 1.646689   0.376494   4.3737 1.221e-05 ***
## e:(Intercept) 0.377269   0.076785   4.9133 8.956e-07 ***
## ---
## Signif. codes: 0 '***' 0.001 '**' 0.01 '*' 0.05 '.' 0.1 ' ' 1
```

By fixing the upper limit, there is a very slight gain in precision for the estimated ED50 (the parameter e), as the standard error becomes a little smaller. In contrast, but in this case of less interest, the precision of the slope parameter b is reduced as the dose 0 is important for estimating the slope. Note that the above comparison between model fits is meant to show how different model choices affect results. However, we want to stress that in practice, ideally, a single model should be chosen up front based on what is known about the experimental design. If this is not feasible, then model averaging is an alternative (see Chapter 6 for more details and examples).

2.2   Analysis of multiple dose-response curves

In this section, we consider two data examples with two and four dose-response curves, respectively. An entire dose-response curve corresponds to a treatment. Ideally, such grouped dose-response data would be analyzed using mixed-effects dose-response models or related techniques. In some cases it may, however, not be feasible to apply such complex methodology.

In both examples below, the main interest lies in comparing treatments in terms of some features of the dose-response curves, which may be captured by model parameters such as LD50 values. In the first example, there are replicated dose-response sub-experiments per treatment. The second example lacks replicated dose-response curves as only one dose-response curve corresponds to one treatment. In such a case there is no way (based on the data alone) to separate random variation between dose-response curves (due to various unobserved differences in the execution of each dose-response sub-experiment) from systematic differences between treatments. Consequently, only weak claims on treatment differences may be made based on such an experimental design.

2.2.1 Toxicity of fluoranthene under different ultraviolet radiation

Wheeler *et al.* (2006) report data from an experiment in which fathead minnow larvae (*Pimephales promelas*) were exposed to fluoranthene, a polycyclic aromatic hydrocarbon, under two different algal densities resulting in different levels of ambient ultraviolet radiation. The two algal concentrations were 0.7 and 1.5 times 10,000 cells. For each algal concentration, four groups of larvae were exposed to fluoranthene concentrations of 5, 10, 20, and 30 μg/L for 4 hours. The number of dead fish larvae out of the total number of larvae was the binomial response of interest. This dose-response experiment was repeated three times (no information for identifying individual experiments was provided). Therefore, we cannot model the experiment-level variation directly in the dose-response model. For now, we note that the assumption of independent binomial responses might be violated.

```
head(fluoranthene)
```

```
##    algalconc conc mortality totalnum
## 1        0.7    5         0       23
## 2        0.7    5         0       19
## 3        0.7    5         0       20
## 4        1.5    5         0       22
## 5        1.5    5         0       25
## 6        1.5    5         0       24
```

We fit a two-parameter log-normal ("log-probit") model to the data although a probit model was originally fitted by Wheeler *et al.* (2006). We prefer the log-normal model as it is only defined for non-negative doses.

```
plot(fluoranthene.LN.2.1, broken = TRUE, type = "all",
     xlim = c(0, 100), ylim = c(0, 1),
     xlab = expression(paste("Concentration (", mu, "g/L)")),
     ylab = "Proportion dead",
     legendPos = c(5, 1))
```

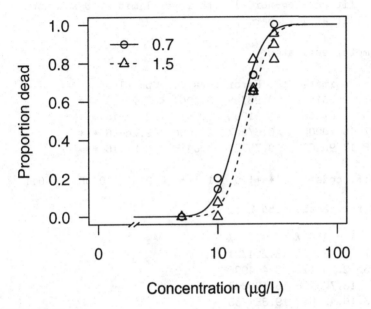

FIGURE 2.3
Two-parameter log-normal model fitted to the dataset **fluoranthene**, one curve for each algal concentration.

```
fluoranthene.LN.2.1 <- drm(mortality/totalnum ~ conc,
                      curveid = algalconc,
                      weights = totalnum,
                      data = fluoranthene,
                      fct = LN.2(),
                      type = "binomial")
```

Note that the second argument in the model specification identifies the individual dose-response curves in the data and here we can only identify the two treatment groups, but not the underlying individual dose-response experiments. Figure 2.3 shows that the fitted dose-response curves capture the trends in the data.

Parameter estimates and the corresponding 95% confidence intervals are shown below.

```
summary(fluoranthene.LN.2.1)
```

```
##
## Model fitted: Log-normal with lower limit at 0 and upper
##      limit at 1 (2 parms)
##
## Parameter estimates:
##
##         Estimate Std. Error t-value   p-value
## b:0.7   2.70147    0.28738  9.4004 < 2.2e-16 ***
## b:1.5   2.87566    0.31085  9.2511 < 2.2e-16 ***
## e:0.7  15.10005    0.67387 22.4080 < 2.2e-16 ***
## e:1.5  17.90466    0.75721 23.6456 < 2.2e-16 ***
## ---
## Signif. codes:  0 '***' 0.001 '**' 0.01 '*' 0.05 '.' 0.1 ' ' 1
```

```
confint(fluoranthene.LN.2.1)
```

```
##              2.5 %    97.5 %
## b:0.7    2.138217  3.264721
## b:1.5    2.266412  3.484906
## e:0.7   13.779295 16.420807
## e:1.5   16.420556 19.388755
```

From the summary it seems that the two slopes could be assumed to be identical, an assumption about parallelism. However, ideally such an assumption should have been imposed before fitting any dose-response model to avoid inflation of standard errors.

As the confidence interval for the two LC50 values are barely overlapping, it could be tempting to claim that the p-value for testing that the two LC50 values are the same is just above 0.05, almost significant. However, in reality the two LC50 values are clearly significantly different. This conclusion may be reached from the direct comparison between the two LC50 values. We use the function compParm() for making comparisons between treatments for a specific model parameter:

```
compParm(fluoranthene.LN.2.1, "e", "-")
```

```
##
## Comparison of parameter 'e'
##
##          Estimate Std. Error t-value p-value
## 0.7-1.5   -2.8046     1.0136 -2.7669 0.00566 **
## ---
## Signif. codes:  0 '***' 0.001 '**' 0.01 '*' 0.05 '.' 0.1 ' ' 1
```

where "e" indicates the model parameter of interest and "-" specifies that comparisons should be in terms of differences (the other option being ratios). The two LC50 values are clearly significantly different.

In an attempt to incorporate the experiment-level variation (as well as any other model misspecification) into the dose-response analysis, we may use the sandwich variance estimator for deriving robust standard errors (see Section A.5 for more details).

```
compParm(fluoranthene.LN.2.1, "e", "-", vcov = sandwich)
```

```
##
## Comparison of parameter 'e'
##
##          Estimate Std. Error t-value  p-value
## 0.7-1.5 -2.80460    0.97744 -2.8693 0.004113 **
## ---
## Signif. codes: 0 '***' 0.001 '**' 0.01 '*' 0.05 '.' 0.1 ' ' 1
```

The conclusion remains the same: there is a clearly significant difference between the two groups in terms of LC50 values (estimated difference: -2.8 (0.977) μg/L, $p = 0.004$).

2.2.2 Toxicity of different types of selenium

In this example, we consider the comparison of four dose-response curves corresponding to four types of selenium (Jeske *et al.*, 2009). Varying numbers of concentrations (5–8, unit unknown) and partly different concentrations of selenium were used. The number of dead flies was recorded. The total number of flies ranged from 63 to 188.

A summary of the dataset is shown below.

```
summary(selenium)
```

```
##       type          conc           total          dead
## Min.   :1.00   Min.   :  0.0   Min.   : 63.0   Min.   :  0.0
## 1st Qu.:2.00   1st Qu.: 25.0   1st Qu.:139.0   1st Qu.: 11.0
## Median :3.00   Median :100.0   Median :146.0   Median : 40.0
## Mean   :2.48   Mean   :190.4   Mean   :142.2   Mean   : 54.4
## 3rd Qu.:3.00   3rd Qu.:300.0   3rd Qu.:153.0   3rd Qu.: 85.0
## Max.   :4.00   Max.   :800.0   Max.   :188.0   Max.   :188.0
```

First, we fit a two-parameter log-logistic model assuming both different slopes and LC50 values for the different types of selenium.

```
selenium.LL.2.1 <- drm(dead/total ~ conc,
                    curveid = type,
                    weights = total,
                    data = selenium,
                    fct = LL.2(),
                    type = "binomial")
```

```
plot(selenium.LL.2.1, type = "all", broken = TRUE,
     xlim = c(0, 10000),
     xlab = "Concentration",
     ylab = "Proportion dead",
     legendPos = c(5, 0.95))
```

The plot of the data with the fitted dose-response curves superimposed shows that the fitted dose-response curves capture the trends in the data quite well (Figure 2.4).

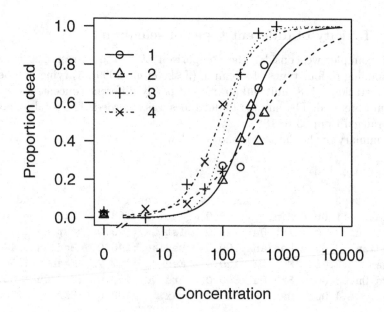

FIGURE 2.4
Two-parameter log-logistic model fitted to the dataset `selenium`. The different line types correspond to the different types of selenium.

Binary and binomial dose-response data 59

The argument `legendPos` was used to specify the position of the legend (more precisely: the top right corner of the box containing the legend).

Next, we fit a two-parameter log-logistic model, but now assuming different slopes and a common LC50 parameter for all four types of selenium.

```
selenium.LL.2.2 <- drm(dead/total~conc,
                        curveid = type,
                        weights = total,
                        data = selenium,
                        fct = LL.2(),
                        type = "binomial",
                        pmodels = list(~factor(type) - 1, ~1))
```

Using the usual formula specification in **R**, we use the argument `pmodels` to specify that there should be different slope parameters b for the different treatments (~`factor(type)` - 1) and a common LC50 for all four treatments (~1).

We can now compare the two model fits using a likelihood ratio test (an approximate chi-square test) by means of the function `anova()`, just like for linear or generalized linear models in **R**.

```
anova(selenium.LL.2.2, selenium.LL.2.1)
```

```
##
## 1st model
## fct:      LL.2()
## pmodels: ~factor(type) - 1, ~1
## 2nd model
## fct:      LL.2()
## pmodels: type (for all parameters)
## ANOVA-like table
##
##           ModelDf  Loglik Df LR value p value
## 1st model       5 -437.99
## 2nd model       8 -376.21  3   123.56       0
```

We can safely conclude that the four LC50 values are not identical ($p < 0.0001$). Jeske *et al.* (2009) reached the same conclusion. The next step is to identify differences between the different types of selenium. The function `EDcomp()` provides all comparisons of LC50 values in terms of ratios:

```
EDcomp(selenium.LL.2.1, c(50, 50))
```

```
##
## Estimated ratios of effect doses
##
```

```
##             Estimate  Std. Error    t-value      p-value
## 1/2:50/50  6.6653e-01  7.8374e-02  -4.2548e+00  2.0922e-05
## 1/3:50/50  2.1072e+00  1.5539e-01   7.1253e+00  1.0387e-12
## 1/4:50/50  2.8405e+00  3.1654e-01   5.8146e+00  6.0771e-09
## 2/3:50/50  3.1614e+00  3.6398e-01   5.9383e+00  2.8804e-09
## 2/4:50/50  4.2617e+00  6.0623e-01   5.3803e+00  7.4368e-08
## 3/4:50/50  1.3480e+00  1.4672e-01   2.3721e+00  1.7689e-02
```

All four types of selenium are significantly different from one another (highest p-value is 0.018). For all types of selenium we calculate both marginal confidence intervals where each single interval has 95% coverage (but this also means that the collection of confidence interval does not have simultaneous 95% coverage) as well as adjusted 95% confidence intervals (with adjustment for simultaneous inference such that the collection of confidence intervals has a 95% coverage). Marginal confidence intervals are obtained using the function ED().

```
ED(selenium.LL.2.1, c(50), interval = "delta")
```

```
##
## Estimated effective doses
##
##          Estimate Std. Error    Lower     Upper
## e:1:50   252.2556    13.8268  225.1555  279.3556
## e:2:50   378.4605    39.3707  301.2953  455.6256
## e:3:50   119.7132     5.9054  108.1389  131.2875
## e:4:50    88.8053     8.6161   71.9180  105.6926
```

To obtain adjusted confidence intervals, we also initially use the function ED() but now supplying the argument multcomp = TRUE to augment the output with a component named EDmultcomp that may be supplied directly to the function glht() in the package *multcomp* (Hothorn et al., 2008). Furthermore, the argument display = FALSE suppresses the printing of marginal confidence intervals, which we have already obtained above.

```
selenium.EDres <- ED(selenium.LL.2.1, c(50),
                     interval = "delta",
                     multcomp = TRUE,
                     display = FALSE)
```

Now we can apply glht() to the object named selenium.EDres. However, to obtain adjusted confidence intervals we can additionally apply confint() directly to the result from glht().

```
confint(glht(selenium.EDres[["EDmultcomp"]]))
```

```
##
##    Simultaneous Confidence Intervals
```

```
##
## Fit: NULL
##
## Quantile = 2.4908
## 95% family-wise confidence level
##
##
## Linear Hypotheses:
##              Estimate lwr      upr
## e:1:50 == 0  252.2556 217.8151 286.6960
## e:2:50 == 0  378.4605 280.3942 476.5267
## e:3:50 == 0  119.7132 105.0039 134.4225
## e:4:50 == 0   88.8053  67.3438 110.2667
```

The resulting adjusted confidence intervals become somewhat wider as compared to the unadjusted marginal ones because of the multiplicity adjustment. In this case the adjustment corresponds to the Bonferroni adjustment as the correlations between estimates are all equal to 0 (Pipper *et al.*, 2012).

It is also possible to obtain all pairwise comparisons of LC50 between the four different types of selenium. Again, we utilize the functionality of *multcomp*: the function call contrMat(1:4, "Tukey") constructs a matrix of all pairwise comparisons of four groups.

```
summary(glht(selenium.EDres[["EDmultcomp"]],
             linfct = contrMat(1:4, "Tukey")))
```

```
##
##   Simultaneous Tests for General Linear Hypotheses
##
## Multiple Comparisons of Means: Tukey Contrasts
##
##
## Linear Hypotheses:
##            Estimate Std. Error z value Pr(>|z|)
## 2 - 1 == 0   126.20      41.73   3.024   0.0111 *
## 3 - 1 == 0  -132.54      15.04  -8.816   <0.001 ***
## 4 - 1 == 0  -163.45      16.29 -10.033   <0.001 ***
## 3 - 2 == 0  -258.75      39.81  -6.499   <0.001 ***
## 4 - 2 == 0  -289.66      40.30  -7.187   <0.001 ***
## 4 - 3 == 0   -30.91      10.45  -2.959   0.0131 *
## ---
## Signif. codes: 0 '***' 0.001 '**' 0.01 '*' 0.05 '.' 0.1 ' ' 1
## (Adjusted p values reported -- single-step method)
```

Using this approach, arbitrary LCxx values may be compared between groups. Moreover, it also works for other types of dose-response data.

3

Count dose-response data

Count data include number of fronds, offspring, juveniles, leaves, or roots, i.e., non-negative integers. In contrast to binomial data, the experimental design imposes no *a priori* upper limit on the counts. In theory, there may be no upper limit although very large counts will be very unlikely. In practice, a limited number of different counts may be observed, but some counts may occur multiple times (with ties). Ideally, counts should be recorded over the same time period in order to be comparable. However, there are ways to adjust for varying durations of the time period. For instance, reproduction data, which are commonly obtained from chronic toxicity tests in ecotoxicology, are often counts of the number of offspring present at the end of the test period (a certain pre-specified time period).

Dose-response analysis of count data is based on statistical models that describe the mean trend on the scale of the counts, not on the scale of the logarithm-transformed mean as would typically be the case for a generalized linear model for count data (McCullagh and Nelder, 1989, Chapter 6). However, the same distributions as used in generalized linear models for counts may be used when fitting dose-response models.

There may be several ways to analyze such count data, depending on the distributional and modeling assumptions one is willing to make (Ritz and Van der Vliet, 2009). In general the closer the chosen distributional assumptions are to the true distributions, which generated the data, the more efficient (i.e., smaller standard errors) the statistical analysis will be. In practice we may not get close to the true distributions, and it will often be a trade-off between more bias in parameter estimates if we are being too confident and choose a quite specific model, and more imprecision (larger estimated standard errors) if we are less picky and choose a model that does not seem fully appropriate (a bias-variance trade-off).

Counts are often assumed to follow a Poisson distribution, although this distribution is not always sufficiently flexible to describe the variation in the count dose-response data (see also Subsection A.2.2.1). The standard deviation of Poisson distributed counts is completely determined by the mean of the distribution; there is no separate parameter for the standard deviation as is the case of the normal distribution. Therefore, it may easily happen that a Poisson distribution does not adequately capture the variation in the observed counts: the counts may exhibit less or more variation than predicted by the Poisson distribution. Excess variation is usually referred to as over-dispersion (e.g., Morgan, 1992, Chapter 6), just as for binomial data. Nevertheless, a Poisson dose-response model may be a good starting point for the analysis.

Apart from the distributional assumptions, dose-response analysis is carried out in much the same way as for continuous dose-response data (Chapter 1), e.g., model checking by means of residuals.

In this chapter, we use the following extension packages:

```
library(drc)
```

```
library(devtools)
install_github("DoseResponse/drcData")
library(drcData)
```

```
library(ggplot2)
```

```
library(lmtest)
```

```
library(multcomp)
```

```
library(dplyr)
```

```
library(sandwich)
```

3.1 Analysis of single dose-response curves

3.1.1 Counting number of fronds

Ritz and Van der Vliet (2009) report dose-response data from a sublethal *Lemna minor* toxicity test where gradual reduction in growth may be observed. Thus, more information may be elicited from this test than from a toxicity test where a binary response is observed (see Chapter 2). Specifically, numbers of fronds from *Lemna minor*, which is an aquatic freshwater plant (common duckweed), were counted for a range of concentrations, which were different dilutions of a metal mining effluent. The dilutions (in percent of the effluent, % v/v) were chosen to ensure that both partial effects and strong inhibitory effects would be observed such that the entire dose-response relationship could be described.

In total 44 plants were examined, corresponding to 10 concentrations including the control. There were 4 replicates for all concentrations except for the control where 8 replicates were used. As seen below, the observed numbers of fronds range from 61–70 in the control group to 29–34 at the highest concentration.

```
head(lemna)
```

```
##   conc frond.num
## 1    0        70
## 2    0        66
## 3    0        61
## 4    0        65
## 5    0        65
## 6    0        61
```

```
lemna %>%
  group_by(conc) %>%
  summarize(min = min(frond.num),
            max = max(frond.num))
```

```
## # A tibble: 10 x 3
##      conc   min   max
##     <dbl> <dbl> <dbl>
## 1  0         61    70
## 2  0.38      64    67
## 3  0.76      54    65
## 4  1.52      55    58
## 5  3.03      50    63
## 6  6.06      49    56
## 7 12.1       41    47
## 8 24.2       37    37
## 9 48.5       31    36
## 10 97        29    34
```

We will fit a Poisson dose-response model, although in our experience, it is not often that a Poisson distribution provides a good description of dose-response count data. In the subsequent subsections, we show how to improve the dose-response model. We will assume that a three-parameter log-logistic model (LL.3()) describes the mean trend in the data adequately.

```
lemna.minor.LL.3 <- drm(frond.num ~ conc,
                        data = lemna,
                        fct = LL.3(),
                        type = "Poisson")
```

It is possible to some extent to validate model assumptions by means of the usual graphical model diagnostics. Below we show a residual plot (using raw residuals will suffice):

```
plot(fitted(lemna.minor.LL.3), residuals(lemna.minor.LL.3),
     xlab = "Fitted values",
     ylab = "Raw residuals")

abline(h=0, lty=2)
```

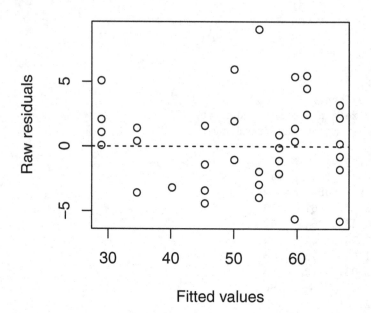

FIGURE 3.1
The residual plot for the three-parameter log-logistic model fitted to the
Lemna minor data.

Based on the residual plot in Figure 3.1 we can conclude that there are no
substantial departures from random scatter (around the y axis). Therefore,
it seems reasonable to assume that a three-parameter log-logistic model will
suffice. We do not look at the standard QQ normal probability plot as it is
not helpful in assessing whether or not the data are Poisson distributed.

The plot of the data with the fitted dose-response curve superimposed is
shown below. Figure 3.2 also supports our initial impression that the three-
parameter log-logistic model describes the data adequately. However, it is
clear that the data hold almost no information about what would happen
for very large concentrations. The assumption about a lower limit of 0 is
crucial as it means that one piece of additional information (not found in the
data!) is incorporated into the model. This consideration is analogous to what
we discussed for continuous dose-response data in Subsection 1.1.5. In case
there are no strong biological reasons for a particular assumption, it may be

```
plot(lemna.minor.LL.3, type = "all", broken = TRUE,
     xlab = "Effluent concentration (% v/v)",
     ylab = "Number of fronds",
     xlim = c(0, 500), ylim = c(0,72),
     conName = "Control", lwd = 2)
```

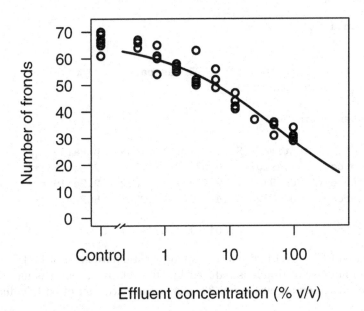

FIGURE 3.2
The fitted three-parameter log-logistic dose-response curve together with the
Lemna minor data.

advisable to fit multiple models such as three- and four-parameter models in
order to appreciate the effect of the absence or presence of such an additional
assumption.

Once we have accepted the model fit as adequately describing the dose-
response data, we can proceed to obtain the estimate of the parameter(s) of
interest, which in this case is a single parameter, namely EC50. It is important to realize that the interpretation of EC50 and indeed any other effective
concentration hinges on the chosen dose-response model function. For the
three-parameter log-logistic model function LL.3(), the estimated EC50 is
the concentration yielding a 50% reduction of the average number of fronds
relative to the average level for the control group, which is the upper limit of
the fitted dose-response curve (corresponding to the estimate of the parameter
d). This definition implicitly assumes that the lower limit of the fitted dose-
response is fixed at 0, corresponding to the plausible biological assumption
that sufficiently high concentrations will result in no growth at all, namely

zero counts. Assuming a non-zero lower limit (LL.4()) may result in a somewhat different result because the estimated EC50 is interpreted relative to the estimated lower and upper limits. In this case, the estimated EC50 becomes approx. 5 times smaller as shown by Van der Vliet and Ritz (2013). This point also applies to continuous dose-response data, but not to binomial dose-response data.

```
summary(lemna.minor.LL.3)
```

```
##
## Model fitted: Log-logistic (ED50 as parameter) with lower
##      limit at 0 (3 parms)
##
## Parameter estimates:
##
##                  Estimate Std. Error t-value   p-value
## b:(Intercept)    0.49207     0.07418  6.6335 3.278e-11 ***
## d:(Intercept)   66.79414     2.59857 25.7042 < 2.2e-16 ***
## e:(Intercept)   56.07520    14.27537  3.9281 8.562e-05 ***
## ---
## Signif. codes: 0 '***' 0.001 '**' 0.01 '*' 0.05 '.' 0.1 ' ' 1
```

The estimated EC50 is 56.1 with a corresponding standard error of 14.3. Thus, the average number of fronds is reduced by 50% relative to an average level of 66.8, i.e., reaching an average of 33.4, at a concentration of 56.1 (effluent % v/v).

As seen previously for continuous data, the generic way to extract EC50 would be to use the function ED(), which may also be used for obtaining other EC values:

```
ED(lemna.minor.LL.3, c(10, 20, 50))
```

```
##
## Estimated effective doses
##
##          Estimate Std. Error
## e:1:10    0.64497    0.46796
## e:1:20    3.35159    1.67765
## e:1:50   56.07520   14.27537
```

The standard errors of the estimated EC10 and also EC20 to some extent are quite large and the corresponding Wald-type 95% confidence interval will have an unrealistic negative lower limit.

```
ED(lemna.minor.LL.3, c(10, 20, 50), interval = "delta")
```

```
##
## Estimated effective doses
```

```
##
##           Estimate Std. Error      Lower      Upper
## e:1:10   0.644967   0.467963  -0.272224   1.562158
## e:1:20   3.351589   1.677654   0.063448   6.639731
## e:1:50  56.075199  14.275369  28.095989  84.054408
```

In principle, it would be possible to reparameterize the model function in such a way that the 95% confidence interval of EC10 is fully contained in the non-negative concentration scale, with a positive lower limit. However, this manoeuvre only conceals the fact that the chosen dose-response model is not capable of eliciting much information on EC10 from the data (possibly because there is almost no information in the data to estimate EC10). Another, possibly improved model may or may not be able to do a better job.

3.1.2 Counting offspring: Modeling hormesis

Bailer and Oris (1997) analyzed data from an experiment where the number of offspring of *C. dubia*, which is a species of water flea used in toxicity testing, was counted after being exposed to different concentrations of waste water for 7 days.

Again, we start out looking at the data. The table below shows that there were 10 replicates for each of five concentrations, one of which is a control group. Next, we can plot the raw data:

```
head(C.dubia)
```

```
##   conc number
## 1    0     27
## 2    0     30
## 3    0     29
## 4    0     31
## 5    0     16
## 6    0     15
```

```
with(C.dubia, table(conc))
```

```
## conc
##    0 1.56 3.12 6.25 12.5
##   10   10   10   10   10
```

Bailer and Oris (1997) fitted a generalized linear model assuming a Poisson distribution and including both linear and quadratic terms of concentrations in order to describe the hormetic effect, which may be inferred from the initial increase in the response for low concentrations, followed by a decreasing response for increasing concentrations (Figure 3.3).

```
plot(number ~ conc, data = C.dubia,
     xlab = "Waste water concentration (%)",
     ylab = "Number of offspring",
     ylim = c(0, 50))
```

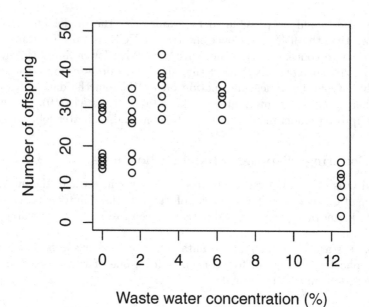

FIGURE 3.3
The scatter plot of the number of offspring as a function of waste water concentration (%) for the *C. dubia* data.

We take a different route by considering dose-response models as defined within the framework of this book. Specifically, we start out fitting a three-parameter log-logistic model assuming that the counts are Poisson distributed (inspired by the previous example); this is an example of an extended generalized linear model where the link function depends on an unknown parameter (in this case the upper limit *d*).

```
C.dubia.LL.3 <- drm(number ~ conc,
                    data = C.dubia,
                    fct = LL.3(),
                    type = "Poisson")
```

The model fit shown in Figure 3.4 (top panel) is not good. For instance, the predicted mean offspring at concentration 0 is not centered among the data points for concentration 0: it has been shifted upwards because of the hormetic effect observed for higher concentrations. Perhaps even more pronounced: the predicted mean number of offspring is too small for the low concentrations that seemed to produce a strong hormetic effect.

As a second attempt we consider the four-parameter Brain-Cousens hormesis model, which may be specified using the function BC.4(). This means we retain the assumption that the lower limit is equal to 0:

```
C.dubia.BC.4 <- drm(number ~ conc,
                    data = C.dubia,
                    fct = BC.4(),
                    type = "Poisson")
```

The fitted dose-response curve is shown in Figure 3.4 (bottom panel). This time the fitted dose-response curve describes the trend in the data very closely (too closely?).

```
plot(C.dubia.LL.3, type = "all", broken = TRUE,
     xlab = "Waste water concentration (%)",
     ylab = "Number of offspring",
     xlim = c(0, 100),
     ylim = c(0, 50))

plot(C.dubia.BC.4, type = "all", broken = TRUE,
     xlab = "Waste water concentration (%)",
     ylab = "Number of offspring",
     xlim = c(0, 100),
     ylim = c(0, 50))
```

Once we have found an appropriate dose-response model, we can take a closer look at the parameter estimates:

```
summary(C.dubia.BC.4)

##
## Model fitted: Brain-Cousens (hormesis) with lower limit fixed
##     at 0 (4 parms)
##
## Parameter estimates:
##
##                 Estimate Std. Error t-value    p-value
## b:(Intercept)  3.83037     0.39251   9.7585 < 2.2e-16 ***
## d:(Intercept) 21.80069     1.38689  15.7191 < 2.2e-16 ***
## e:(Intercept)  7.60327     0.61601  12.3427 < 2.2e-16 ***
## f:(Intercept)  4.03279     0.88706   4.5462 5.462e-06 ***
## ---
## Signif. codes: 0 '***' 0.001 '**' 0.01 '*' 0.05 '.' 0.1 ' ' 1
```

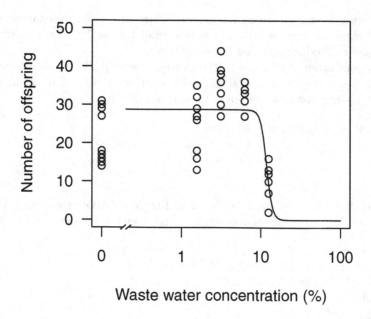

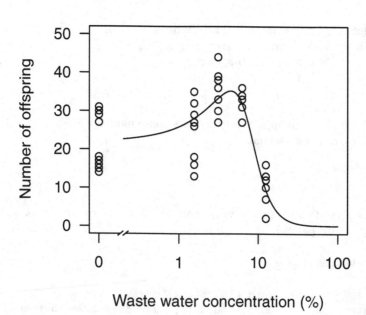

FIGURE 3.4
The fitted three-parameter log-logistic and four-parameter Brain-Cousens hormesis models shown together with the *C. dubia* data.

The parameter f quantifies the extent of the hormetic effect in the sense that the more positive this parameter is, the larger is the hormesis peak. The parameter f is significantly different from 0, implying that there is a substantial hormetic effect. Bailer and Oris (1997) reached the same conclusion based on a quadratic generalized linear model.

The `summary` output does not provide any estimate of EC50. In contrast to the four-parameter log-logistic model, the parameter e has lost its interpretation as EC50 in the hormesis models. Therefore, to estimate EC50, we use the function `ED()`:

```
ED(C.dubia.BC.4, 50)
```

```
##
## Estimated effective doses
##
##         Estimate Std. Error
## e:1:50  11.7863     0.5086
```

For hormesis models and biphasic dose-response models in general, it may be possible to estimate EC values for both phases, i.e., corresponding to effects to the left and right of the peak. For instance, we can estimate EC-10 and EC-20 as follows (notice the use of the additional argument `bound = FALSE`, which switches off checking if the specified effect levels lie between 0 and 100):

```
ED(C.dubia.BC.4, c(-10, -20), bound = FALSE)
```

```
##
## Estimated effective doses
##
##          Estimate Std. Error
## e:1:-10  8.09294    0.46267
## e:1:-20  7.61867    0.49695
```

Actually, EC-10 and EC-20 turn out to be almost as precisely determined from the data as is EC50 (with comparable standard errors), reflecting that these estimates are within the concentration range where actual concentrations are found in the data.

3.1.3 More counting offspring: Varying observation periods

Delignette-Muller *et al.* (2014b) reported reproduction data for *Daphnia Magna* exposed to different concentrations of the insecticide chlordane ($\mu g/L$). There are 6 concentrations, including one control group, and 10 replicates per concentration. Specifically, numbers of offspring were counted over an observation period of 21 days. If a daphnia died during the 21, days the number of offspring until death was counted. For daphnias, the duration of the observation period was observed. We start out by looking at the data.

```
head(chlordan)
```

```
##   replicate conc repro time
## 1         1 0.00   125 21.0
## 2         1 0.18    89 21.0
## 3         1 0.73    90 21.0
## 4         1 1.82    42 21.0
## 5         1 2.90    29 21.0
## 6         1 7.00    10 11.5
```

As a first naïve approach we can fit a three-parameter log-logistic model, assuming Poisson distributed counts but ignoring the duration of the observation periods. This model describes the total number of offspring over 21 days.

```
chlordan.LL.3 <- drm(repro ~ conc,
                     data = chlordan,
                     fct = LL.3(),
                     type = "Poisson")
```

The residual plot shown in Figure 3.5 looks reasonable. Likewise, the fitted dose-response model seems to describe the trend in the data adequately (Figure 3.6).

Now we can take a look at the summary output:

```
summary(chlordan.LL.3)
```

```
##
## Model fitted: Log-logistic (ED50 as parameter) with lower
##     limit at 0 (3 parms)
##
## Parameter estimates:
##
##                   Estimate Std. Error t-value   p-value
## b:(Intercept)     1.089500   0.070639  15.423 < 2.2e-16 ***
## d:(Intercept)   113.666336   2.984324  38.088 < 2.2e-16 ***
## e:(Intercept)     1.615563   0.127838  12.638 < 2.2e-16 ***
## ---
## Signif. codes: 0 '***' 0.001 '**' 0.01 '*' 0.05 '.' 0.1 ' ' 1
```

The estimated EC50 is 1.62 (0.13). The estimated average total reproduction over 21 days in the control group is 114 (2.98) offspring.

Using the `confint` method we find the 95% confidence interval for EC50.

```
confint(chlordan.LL.3)
```

```
##                     2.5 %     97.5 %
## b:(Intercept)   0.9510493    1.22795
## d:(Intercept) 107.8171683  119.51550
## e:(Intercept)   1.3650065    1.86612
```

```
plot(fitted(chlordan.LL.3), residuals(chlordan.LL.3))
abline(h=0, lty=2)
```

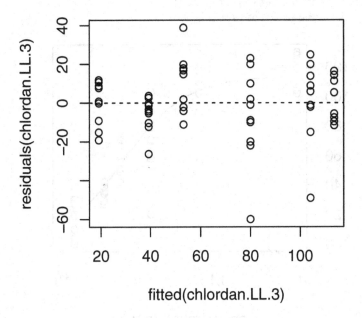

fitted(chlordan.LL.3)

FIGURE 3.5
The residual plot for the three-parameter log-logistic model fitted to the
chlordan dataset.

As already mentioned, there is some imbalance in durations of observation
periods, which implies that counts even obtained at the same concentration
may not be comparable as they were recorded over varying time periods.
Specifically, the distribution of durations of observation periods looks like this:

```
with(chlordan, table(time))

## time
##  2.5  9.5 11.5 14.5 17.5 18.5 20.5   21
##    1    2    3    1    1    9    1   42
```

The above dose-response model did not incorporate this imbalance and, hence,
it may be seen as a misspecified model (as the distributional assumptions are
partly misspecified). Ideally, such imbalance should be taken into account in
the statistical analysis in order to reduce bias in the estimates.

One approach is to fit a three-parameter log-logistic model but use the durations of observation periods as weights; this means that numbers of offspring

```
plot(chlordan.LL.3,
     broken = TRUE,
     type = "all",
     xlim = c(0, 10),
     xlab = "Concentration (mu g/L)",
     ylab = "Number of offspring")
```

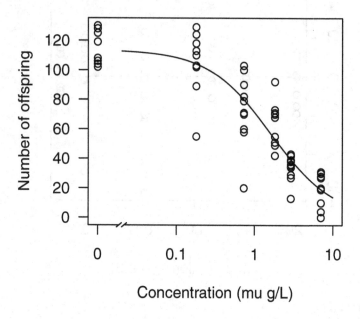

FIGURE 3.6
The fitted three-parameter log-logistic dose-response curve to the `chlordan`
dataset shown together with the raw data.

are scaled by their durations. This again means that the average number of
offspring *per day* for a given concentration is modeled. In particular, the parameter d can be interpreted as the average number of offspring per day in the
unexposed control group. However, it is important to stress that the scaling
or normalization by duration is taken care of by the model.

   The weighted Poisson model is fitted as follows using the argument
`weights`:

```
chlordan.LL.3.we <- drm(repro ~ conc,
                        data = chlordan,
                        fct = LL.3(),
                        type = "Poisson",
                        weights = time)
```

The resulting **summary** output is obtained here:

```
summary(chlordan.LL.3.we)
```

```
##
## Model fitted: Log-logistic (ED50 as parameter) with lower
##     limit at 0 (3 parms)
##
## Parameter estimates:
##
##               Estimate Std. Error t-value   p-value
## b:(Intercept) 0.929859   0.065783  14.135 < 2.2e-16 ***
## d:(Intercept) 5.544291   0.146147  37.936 < 2.2e-16 ***
## e:(Intercept) 1.758823   0.151862  11.582 < 2.2e-16 ***
## ---
## Signif. codes: 0 '***' 0.001 '**' 0.01 '*' 0.05 '.' 0.1 ' ' 1
```

The estimated EC50 is now 1.76 (0.15). The estimated average daily reproduction rate in the control group is 5.54 (0.146) offspring.

Looking at Figure 3.6 (note in particular the variation in the mid-range of concentrations), we may suspect that model misspecification is not only due to the varying durations but also caused by over-dispersion. Therefore, another approach would be to fit a negative-binomial model. Such a model may be specified using **type = "negbin2"**; there is also the option **"negbin1"** for a slightly different model (Delignette-Muller *et al.*, 2014b).

```
chlordan.LL.3.nb.we <-drm(repro ~ conc,
                          data = chlordan,
                          fct = LL.3(),
                          type = "negbin2",
                          weight = time)
```

Again, we look at the summary output, which should be interpreted in exactly the same way as for the weighted Poisson model:

```
summary(chlordan.LL.3.nb.we)
```

```
##
## Model fitted: Log-logistic (ED50 as parameter) with lower
##     limit at 0 (3 parms)
##
## Parameter estimates:
##
##               Estimate Std. Error t-value   p-value
## b:(Intercept)  0.91769    0.11430  8.0291 9.349e-16 ***
## d:(Intercept)  5.57532    0.27033 20.6242 < 2.2e-16 ***
## e:(Intercept)  1.68993    0.27040  6.2498 4.111e-10 ***
## 0:(Intercept) -2.18109    0.28539 -7.6426 2.130e-14 ***
```

```
## ---
## Signif. codes: 0 '***' 0.001 '**' 0.01 '*' 0.05 '.' 0.1 ' ' 1

confint(chlordan.LL.3.nb.we)

##                     2.5 %      97.5 %
## b:(Intercept)   0.6936773    1.141707
## d:(Intercept)   5.0454867    6.105160
## e:(Intercept)   1.1599602    2.219908
## O:(Intercept)  -2.7404380   -1.621742
```

Slightly different parameter estimates are obtained, but the standard errors are almost twice as large as compared to the Poisson model. The parameter, O, appearing in the summary output is $\exp(\omega)$ in Equation (A.8) in Section A.2.2.2.

One last alternative approach would be to adjust for model misspecification in terms of the assumed distribution (while still assuming that the dose-response model function is correctly specified) by replacing the default naïve standard errors by robust standard errors (see Section A.5).

```
coeftest(chlordan.LL.3, vcov. = sandwich)

##
## t test of coefficients:
##
##                   Estimate Std. Error t value   Pr(>|t|)
## b:(Intercept)      1.08950    0.17078  6.3795  3.413e-08 ***
## d:(Intercept)    113.66634    4.25420 26.7186  < 2.2e-16 ***
## e:(Intercept)      1.61556    0.25454  6.3470  3.862e-08 ***
## ---
## Signif. codes: 0 '***' 0.001 '**' 0.01 '*' 0.05 '.' 0.1 ' ' 1
```

This approach results in exactly the same parameter estimates as for the unweighted Poisson model but with modified standard errors, which are almost twice as large. Indeed, the results are similar to the results from the fitted negative binomial model.

In terms of point estimates and 95% confidence intervals, the above results for the models taking the weights into account are very similar to the results originally reported by Delignette-Muller *et al.* (2014a) but obtained using a much more complex Bayesian approach.

3.2 Analysis of multiple dose-response curves

In this section, we consider one data example with two dose-response curves and an external control group. An entire dose-response curve corresponds to a single treatment, but as there are no replicated dose-response curves, systematic treatment differences cannot be separated from random variation between dose-response curves. We can still compare treatment groups, as you will see below, but it will take additional arguments (independent of the dose-response data) and information to rule out confounding.

3.2.1 Counting bacteria colonies: Wadley's problem

Trajstman (1989) describes a laboratory experiment on isolation of *Mycobacterium bovis* (*M. bovis*) colonies, which cause bovine tuberculosis. In short, *M. bovis* is detected from bovine tissues grown on culture plates if *M. bovis* colonies appear after some time. As *M. bovis* colonies are slow growing, contaminating bacteria may overgrow the cultures. Decontaminants may be used for killing contaminating bacteria. However, the dose is important to avoid that *M. bovis* are also killed while ensuring uncontaminated plates. In this experiment the performance of two decontaminants, oxalic acid and 1-hexadecylpyridium chloride (HPC), was compared. The dataset decontaminants is shown below.

```
head(decontaminants)

##    conc count group
## 1 0.75     2   hpc
## 2 0.75     4   hpc
## 3 0.75     8   hpc
## 4 0.75     9   hpc
## 5 0.75    10   hpc
## 6 0.75     1   hpc

summary(decontaminants)

##       conc              count          group
## Min.   :0.0000   Min.   : 0.00   hpc   :69
## 1st Qu.:0.0050   1st Qu.:18.00   oxalic:59
## Median :0.0750   Median :33.00
## Mean   :0.5503   Mean   :32.27
## 3rd Qu.:0.3750   3rd Qu.:46.00
## Max.   :5.0000   Max.   :80.00
```

Ten plates were used at each level of decontaminant concentration. Separately, 20 plates without any decontaminant were used for the control experiment. The numbers of colonies on the plates were counted.

We revisit the analysis of the data that was carried out by Morgan and Smith (1992). However, instead of separate models per decontaminant, we fit a joint model including both decontaminants as well as the control group, which was common to the two groups. Specifically, we use the argument pmodels to indicate that the parameter d is shared among the three groups ($\sim$1), whereas the parameters b and d should be different between the two groups ($\sim$group-1). Note that this model specification is only possible because the data have been arranged in such a way that the control group has been merged with one of the two other groups (it does not matter which one). Following the original analysis we fit a three-parameter Weibull type 1 model. This model fitting is an example of Wadley's problem (Finney, 1971, Chapter 10).

```
decon.W1.3.po <- drm(count ~ conc,
                     curveid = group,
                     data = decontaminants,
                     fct = W1.3(),
                     type = "Poisson",
                     pmodels = list(~ group-1, ~ 1, ~ group-1))
```

```
decon.summary <- decontaminants %>%
  group_by(group, conc) %>%
  summarise(mean.count = mean(count),
            sd2.count=var(count))
```

```
plot(sd2.count ~ mean.count, data = decon.summary,
     ylim = c(0, 160),
     xlab = "Average count",
     ylab = "Squared standard deviation")
```

```
abline(a = 0, b = 1, lty = 2)
```

The plot of average counts versus squared empirical standard deviations in Figure 3.7 indicates that the variation increases more with increasing average counts than can be explained by the Poisson distribution (points tend to be above the 45° reference line), i.e., over-dispersion is present.

Therefore, we expect that the standard errors of parameter estimates reported in the summary output below are too small as the Poisson model is not able to incorporate all variation in the counts:

```
summary(decon.W1.3.po)
```

```
##
## Model fitted: Weibull (type 1) with lower limit at 0 (3 parms)
##
## Parameter estimates:
##
##                   Estimate Std. Error t-value   p-value
## b:grouphpc        0.773346   0.051621 14.9813 < 2.2e-16 ***
## b:groupoxalic     0.371221   0.039024  9.5127 < 2.2e-16 ***
```

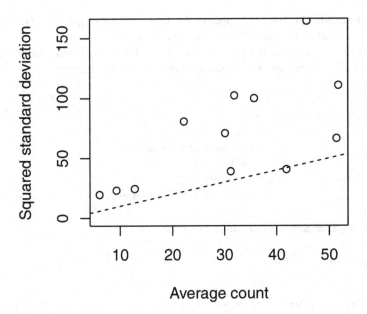

FIGURE 3.7
Average counts versus squared empirical standard deviations per concentration per decontaminant for the `decontaminants` dataset. The broken line corresponds to the variation predicted by the Poisson distribution.

```
## d:(Intercept) 49.848286   1.218586 40.9066 < 2.2e-16 ***
## e:grouphpc     0.268028   0.017093 15.6803 < 2.2e-16 ***
## e:groupoxalic  1.498828   0.238817  6.2761 3.473e-10 ***
## ---
## Signif. codes:  0 '***' 0.001 '**' 0.01 '*' 0.05 '.' 0.1 ' ' 1
```

One way to take over-dispersion into account is by using robust standard errors.

```
coeftest(decon.W1.3.po, vcov = sandwich)
##
## t test of coefficients:
##
##                  Estimate Std. Error t value  Pr(>|t|)
## b:grouphpc       0.773346   0.107492  7.1945 5.387e-11 ***
## b:groupoxalic    0.371221   0.090580  4.0983 7.498e-05 ***
## d:(Intercept)   49.848286   2.506653 19.8864 < 2.2e-16 ***
## e:grouphpc       0.268028   0.039689  6.7531 5.102e-10 ***
## e:groupoxalic    1.498828   0.508578  2.9471  0.003839 **
## ---
## Signif. codes:  0 '***' 0.001 '**' 0.01 '*' 0.05 '.' 0.1 ' ' 1
```

The robust standard errors are approximately 2–3 times larger than the naïve standard errors shown in the above summary output.

An alternative approach would be to retain the three-parameter Weibull type 1 model but replace the Poisson distribution by a negative binomial distribution:

```
decon.W1.3.nb <- drm(count ~ conc,
                     curveid = group,
                     data = decontaminants,
                     fct = W1.3(),
                     type = "negbin2",
                     pmodels = list(~ group-1, ~ 1, ~ group-1))
```

The resulting summary output looks like this:

```
summary(decon.W1.3.nb)

##
## Model fitted: Weibull (type 1) with lower limit at 0 (3 parms)
##
## Parameter estimates:
##
##                   Estimate Std. Error t-value    p-value
## b:grouphpc        0.777719   0.083595  9.3034 < 2.2e-16 ***
## b:groupoxalic     0.368470   0.061458  5.9955 2.029e-09 ***
## d:(Intercept)    50.014470   1.988664 25.1498 < 2.2e-16 ***
## e:grouphpc        0.264038   0.026979  9.7868 < 2.2e-16 ***
## e:groupoxalic     1.463080   0.379882  3.8514 0.0001174 ***
## 0:(Intercept)     0.505370   0.208863  2.4196 0.0155366 *
## ---
## Signif. codes: 0 '***' 0.001 '**' 0.01 '*' 0.05 '.' 0.1 ' ' 1
```

We see the same picture: standard errors increased as compared to the Poisson model, but less dramatically this time: only around a factor 2. The fitted dose-response curves based on the negative binomial model are shown in Figure 3.8.

The potency of two decontaminants may be compared in terms of the ratio of their EC50 values using the function EDcomp():

```
EDcomp(decon.W1.3.nb, c(50, 50), interval = "delta")

##
## Estimated ratios of effect doses
##
##                    Estimate   Lower   Upper
## hpc/oxalic:50/50    0.30459 0.11155 0.49763
```

```
plot(decon.W1.3.nb, broken = TRUE, type = "all",
    xlim = c(0, 10),
    xlab = "Concentration (% w/v)",
    ylab = "Colonies")
```

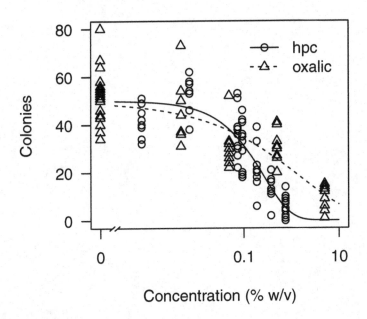

FIGURE 3.8
Three-parameter Weibull type 1 model fitted to the dataset `decontaminants`.

There is a significant difference in the potency of the two decontaminants ($p <$ 0.0001). Moreover, the decontaminant HPC is approximately 0.305 (0.112, 0.498) times as potent as oxalic acid.

4

Multinomial dose-response data

A multinomial response is usually ordinal, providing a more detailed picture of gradual change than the one offered by a binary response. A prominent example is various severity scores ranging from unaffected/alive through one or more stages of being partially affected to 100% affected/dead.

There exists very little work on the statistical analysis of multinomial dose-response data. Some authors have used general modeling approaches for multinomial data (Finney, 1971, pp. 220-226; Morgan, 1992, pp. 119–12), whereas others have proposed novel approaches specifically for dose-response data (Fox and Landis, 2016).

We will take a different, pragmatic and practical approach towards analysis of multinomial dose-response data, exploiting that such data may be analyzed through a series of models fitted to suitably derived binomial dose-response data. Specifically, if there are K categories in the multinomial dose-response data, then $K - 1$ models for binomial dose-response data need to be fitted (there may be several ways of doing this); the examples will demonstrate how to do this in practice. Admittedly, this approach is an approximation: The loss in efficiency from not having a joint model for the multinomial data, but repeatedly fitting models to derived binomial data, however, seems to be small in most cases (Begg and Gray, 1984).

One key advantage of fitting multiple models to binomial dose-response data is that it becomes easier to interpret the results. Another advantage is that over-dispersion, which can also occur for multinomial data, may be dealt with the same way as for binomial data. One disadvantage may possibly be that the obtained results are less parsimonious, but models for multinomial data also yield results that are more challenging to interpret.

Below we consider two textbook examples with trichotomous dose-response data, but the approach also works for multinomial data with more categories.

In this chapter we use the following extension packages:

```
library(drc)

library(devtools)
install_github("doseResponse/drcData")
library(drcData)

install_github("SigneMJensen/mmmVcov")
```

```
library(mmmVcov)

library(multcomp)

library(dplyr)
```

4.1 Trichotomous data

4.1.1 Insecticide residues

Finney (1971, pp. 223–226) analyzed data from an experiment investigating the effect of residues found in alfalfa plants that were sprayed with one of two preparations (Standard vs. Test) of the insecticide guthion in varying doses (μg (Standard) and ml (Test)). For each dose, 50 insects were exposed to the residue for 17 hours. Then the number of alive, moribund, and dead insects were counted.

```
guthion
```

```
##    trt dose alive moribund dead total
## 1    S 20.0    44        1    5    50
## 2    S 35.0    28        1   21    50
## 3    S 45.0     8        7   35    50
## 4    T  1.0    37        1   12    50
## 5    T  1.5    20        2   28    50
## 6    T  2.0     8        6   36    50
```

We fit the two-parameter log-logistic model to binomial data obtained from the multinomial data by merging the two categories "alive" and "moribund" into a single category while retaining the category "dead." The following analysis compares "dead" to "moribund" and "alive" combined:

```
guthion.LL.2.am <- drm(dead/total ~ dose,
                       curveid = trt,
                       weights = total,
                       data = guthion,
                       fct = LL.2(),
                       type = "binomial")
```

Estimated LC50 values and their ratio are obtained as in the previous chapters using the functions ED() and EDcomp()

```
ED(guthion.LL.2.am, c(50))
```

```
##
## Estimated effective doses
##
##          Estimate Std. Error
## e:S:50 36.891558    1.887823
## e:T:50  1.432554    0.083677
```

```
EDcomp(guthion.LL.2.am, c(50, 50), interval = "delta")
```

```
##
## Estimated ratios of effect doses
##
##              Estimate  Lower   Upper
## S/T:50/50      25.752 21.833 29.672
```

The estimated relative potency is close to the one obtained by Finney (1971, p. 226) (the difference most likely due to different estimation procedures). Next, we fit the two-parameter log-logistic model to binomial data obtained by merging the neighbouring categories "moribund" and "dead" into a single category while retaining the category "alive" unchanged. In general, you may want to merge more and more categories starting from 100% affected/dead to compare decreasing accumulated severity to alive. Or you start from unaffected/alive and include more and more severe stages step by step. The following analysis compares "moribund" and "dead" combined to "alive":

```
guthion.LL.2.dm <- drm((moribund+dead)/total ~ dose,
                    curveid = trt,
                    weights = total,
                    data = guthion,
                    fct = LL.2(),
                    type = "binomial")
```

Estimated LC50 values and their ratio are obtained as before:

```
ED(guthion.LL.2.dm, c(50))
```

```
##
## Estimated effective doses
##
##          Estimate Std. Error
## e:S:50 33.908787    1.552187
## e:T:50  1.324984    0.066308
```

```
EDcomp(guthion.LL.2.dm, c(50, 50), interval = "delta")
```

```
##
## Estimated ratios of effect doses
```

```
##
##                 Estimate  Lower   Upper
## S/T:50/50        25.592  22.190  28.994
```

Again, the estimated relative potency is close to the one obtained by Finney (1971, p. 226). Figure 4.1 also shows that the two model fits are quite similar in terms of differences between the two groups, reflecting that the "moribund" category contains only little information.

```
plot(guthion.LL.2.am, broken = TRUE, type = "all",
     xlim = c(0, 1000),
     ylim = c(0, 1),
     xlab = "Dose",
     ylab = "Proportion affected")

plot(guthion.LL.2.dm, add = TRUE, col = "gray",
     xlim = c(0, 1000),
     legend = FALSE)
```

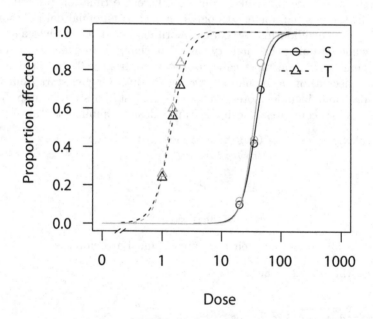

FIGURE 4.1
Two-parameter log-logistic models fitted to binomial data obtained from the dataset `guthion`. Black lines for the analysis of "dead" vs. "alive" and "moribund" combined, grey lines for the analysis of "dead" and "moribund" combined vs. "alive."

Moreover, the fitted binomial dose-response models have fairly similar estimated slope parameters in both model fits (keeping in mind the narrow range of the doses applied: 1, 45):

```
coef(summary(guthion.LL.2.am))[1:2, ]
```

```
##          Estimate Std. Error    t-value      p-value
## b:S -3.768548  0.7123614 -5.290220 1.221692e-07
## b:T -3.051117  0.6568528 -4.645054 3.399877e-06
```

```
coef(summary(guthion.LL.2.dm))[1:2, ]
```

```
##          Estimate Std. Error    t-value      p-value
## b:S -4.365964  0.7367935 -5.925628 3.111063e-09
## b:T -3.850136  0.7031664 -5.475427 4.364577e-08
```

(using square brackets to choose the first two rows containing the estimated slopes). This indicates that the proportional odds assumption would be appropriate for these multinomial data (e.g., Morgan, 1992, p. 120). Note that if we had instead fitted Weibull type 2 models (using W2.2()) we could have assessed in the same way if a proportional hazards assumption would have been appropriate. However, in contrast to the analysis reported by Finney (1971, pp. 223–226), the approach based on analyzing several binomial datasets does not rely on any proportional odds assumption; we prefer this approach. If a single pooled estimate of the relative potency is of interest and possibly warranted (as in this case) then it may be derived by averaging the estimates from the binomial model fits as shown below.

We use the function mjust() from the GitHub package *mmmVcov* to estimate the variance-covariance matrix of the two relative potencies, i.e., to obtain estimated standard errors and, more importantly, the estimated correlation between the two estimated relative potencies (which are estimated from two marginal model fits, not from a joint model fit). This is possible using **R** but, to our knowledge, not in any other statistical software (Jensen and Ritz, 2015).

```
relPot.pooled <- mjust(list(guthion.LL.2.am, guthion.LL.2.dm),
                       list("e_S/e_T", "e_S/e_T"), seType = "san")
```

```
relPot.pooled[["covar"]]
```

```
##            [,1]      [,2]
## [1,] 0.4024401 0.5548167
## [2,] 0.5548167 1.8861332
```

```
confint(glht(parm(relPot.pooled[["coef"]][,1],
             relPot.pooled[["covar"]]),
        linfct = matrix(c(0.5, 0.5), 1, 2)))
```

```
##
##    Simultaneous Confidence Intervals
##
## Fit: NULL
##
## Quantile = 1.96
## 95% family-wise confidence level
##
##
## Linear Hypotheses:
##         Estimate lwr      upr
## 1 == 0 25.6721  23.8656  27.4786
```

The argument seType = "san" implies that robust standard errors and correlations are estimated (Jensen and Ritz, 2018). Once the variance-covariance matrix has been estimated (and stored under the name relPot.pooled) the functions glht() and parm() from the package *multcomp* may be used to calculate the average of the two estimates (specified using linfct = matrix(c(0.5, 0.5), 1, 2)) and the corresponding estimated standard error. Finally, confint() produces the associated confidence interval (95% by default). Note that the confidence interval is narrower than the two confidence intervals derived from the binomial dose-response models.

4.1.2   Effect of two arboviruses on chicken embryos

Morgan (1992) discusses a trichotomous multinomial data example where chicken embryos were exposed to increasing doses of an arbovirus (PFA/embryo) in order to investigate the potency of the virus. The experiment was carried out for two different types of arbovirus (below denoted "FP" and "T," respectively). Initially there were 20 embryos per dose, but a few embryos died of other reasons in the first few days. After 18 days each embryo was assessed and categorised as not deformed, deformed, or dead (three categories). The entire dataset is shown below.

arbovirus

```
##     dose total dead def trt
## 1      3    17    3   1  FP
## 2     18    19    4   1  FP
## 3     30    19    8   2  FP
## 4     90    20   17   1  FP
## 5      3    19    1   0   T
## 6     20    19    2   0   T
## 7   2400    15    4   9   T
## 8  88000    19    9  10   T
## 9      0    18    1   0   T
```

We follow the same steps as in the previous subsection: First we fit a two-parameter log-logistic model to binomial data obtained by merging the not deformed and deformed categories into a single category:

```
arbovirus.LL.2.dead <- drm(dead/total ~ dose,
                    curveid = trt,
                    weights = total,
                    data = arbovirus,
                    fct = LL.2(),
                    type = "binomial")
```

Next we fit the model where binomial data were obtained by merging deformed and dead categories:

```
arbovirus.LL.2.alive <- drm((def+dead)/total ~ dose,
                    curveid = trt,
                    weights = total,
                    data = arbovirus,
                    fct = LL.2(),
                    type = "binomial")
```

Figure 4.2 shows the fitted dose-response curves with the data. It is apparent that the estimated slope coefficients are different between the two analyses, i.e., the proportional odds assumption seems not appropriate. We proceed to summarize the model fits one by one. First the results for the analysis of dead vs. deformed+alive:

```
EDcomp(arbovirus.LL.2.dead, c(50, 50), interval = "delta",
       reverse = TRUE)

##
## Estimated ratios of effect doses
##
##              Estimate  Lower   Upper
## T/FP:50/50    1284.5  -1007.2  3576.1
```

We use the argument **reverse = TRUE** to reverse the calculation to have the reciprocal relative potency estimated (showing how much more potent arbovirus FP is than arbovirus T); by default it would be the other way around. The estimated relative potency of arbovirus FP relative to arbovirus T is 1284. In other words the arbovirus FR is approx. 1300 times more potent than the arbovirus T in killing chicken embryos.

For the second analysis where "deformed" and "dead" were merged we get the following results:

```
plot(arbovirus.LL.2.dead, broken = TRUE,
    xlim = c(0, 1000000),
    ylim = c(0, 1),
    xlab = "Dose (plaque-forming assay per embryo)",
    ylab = "Proportion affected",
    legendPos = c(7, 1))

plot(arbovirus.LL.2.alive, add = TRUE, col = "gray",
    legend = FALSE)
```

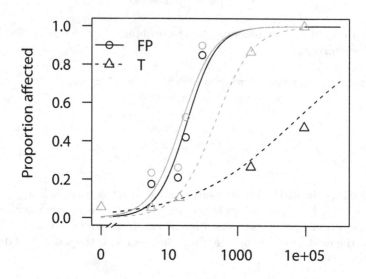

FIGURE 4.2
Two-parameter log-logistic models fitted to binomial data derived from the dataset arbovirus. Black lines for the analysis of dead vs. alive+deformed, grey lines for the analysis of dead+deformed vs. alive.

```
EDcomp(arbovirus.LL.2.alive, c(50, 50), interval = "delta",
       reverse = TRUE)
```

```
##
## Estimated ratios of effect doses
##
##              Estimate   Lower    Upper
## T/FP:50/50     9.4238  -2.7513  21.5988
```

The estimated relative potency of arbovirus T relative to arbovirus FP is 9.424. The arbovirus FP is approximately 10 times more potent than the arbovirus T in being harmful to chicken embryos.

Due to the small sample size in general and the dose range of arbovirus T not capturing the full response range, the 95% confidence intervals of the relative potencies have lower limits below 0, which is not meaningful as relative potencies are by definition positive. These lower limits should be truncated at 0, indicating that there is only little information in the dose-response data for estimating relative potencies.

5

Time-to-event-response data

Time-to-event-response data, which are a special type of time-to-event data, occur frequently in biology, ecology, seed science, and toxicology as the result of planned experiments.

A time to event (also called an event time) is the time it takes until some well-defined event happens (e.g., a plant flowering or a seed germinating). However, the event of interest is usually not observed exactly at the time point where it took place. This feature usually reflects limitations in the practical management of experiments and it is only possible to determine timing of events to have taken place in a certain time interval. Our way of collecting or observing data leads to a grouping of the time-to-event data according to the monitoring interval (although the event itself can happen at any time, in continuous time). Moreover, the event of interest need not occur at all during the time course of the experiment. This feature is commonly referred to as right censoring: the experiment had been terminated before the event would possibly have happened or the event was rendered impossible during the experiment. Morgan (1992) already pointed out these characteristics but it seems not to have had much influence on the data analysis in practice, possibly because of lack of suitable statistical software.

For instance, in germination experiments, time to seed germination is one outcome of interest. Seeds may only be inspected once a day or week and once a seed has germinated, the only information obtained is that the event (seed germination) took place somewhere between the last and the present inspection. Furthermore, some seeds may remain dormant for the entire duration of the experiment or some seeds may have been eaten or rotted away during the experiment.

General time-to-event data are often analyzed by means of semi- or non-parametric survival analysis methods. In contrast, we will only use fully parametric models to analyze time-to-event-response, as they are equally flexible and more easily provide relevant and interpretable parameter estimates. There has been a long tradition for analysis of germination data by means of logistic and nonlinear regression techniques although these approaches have some shortcomings (Morgan, 1992; Ritz *et al.*, 2013b). In particular, these methods may lead to too small estimated standard errors for parameter estimates of interest (e.g., t_{50}) as these techniques do not account for the loss of information due to grouping and right censoring.

Models that are more appropriate need to incorporate time-to-event data, which are both grouped and right-censored. However, only recently such models have been developed and, indeed, implemented in **R** in a general framework, which may be useful for other types of time-to-event-response data, not only germination data (Ritz *et al.*, 2013b).

The key insight linking the present chapter with the previous chapters on modeling of continuous, binomial, count, and trichotomous dose-response data is that cumulative distribution functions are special cases of dose-response model functions with a few restrictions imposed (the time elapsed since the beginning of the experiment is "the dose"). In practice, it means we have nearly the same flexibility for modeling time-to-event-response data as for any other type of dose-response data.

For convenience, we assume that the experiment begins at time 0. We formulate the statistical model in terms of the cumulative distribution function F, which for each time point $t \geq 0$ describes the fraction of events that took place between time 0 and time t. By definition F is 0 at time 0 and $F(t)$ approaches a fraction $d \leq 1$ as more and more time elapses. If $d < 1$ then we will assume that F has a jump and reaches 1 at infinity, that is $F(\infty) = 1$ (otherwise F is not a cumulative distribution function). This modeling assumption implies that there is possibly a proportion of events (equal to $1 - d$) that will not be observed to happen during the experiment (regardless of the duration of the experiment). In each application, it has to be judged if this is a reasonable assumption.

We consider model parameterizations of the cumulative distribution function that ensures both $F(0) = 0$ and convenient biological interpretations (Ritz *et al.*, 2013b). This parallels the dose-response modeling approach from the previous chapters. A commonly used model is the three-parameter log-logistic model:

$$F(t) = \frac{d}{1 + \exp[b\{\log(t) - \log(t_{50})\}]} = \frac{d}{1 + \left(\frac{t}{t_{50}}\right)^b}, \qquad (5.1)$$

which is identical to the three-parameter log-logistic function introduced previously, but now as a function of time (t) instead of dose. The interpretation of the slope parameter b is unaltered. The parameter t_{50} is the time point where 50% of the events have happened, that is, by definition, it is relative to the maximum proportion d observed during the experiment. Thus, the parameter t_{50} has the same interpretation in terms of a halfway reduction relative to the achievable maximum as has the ED50 for continuous data. In particular, this means that t_{50} only corresponds to the median event time in case $d = 1$, in which case $F(t_{50}) = 0.5$. In general, this will not hold for the model defined by Equation (5.1). In the general case, t_{50} corresponds to the $100d/2$ percentile in the distribution of event times. See Section A.2.3 for more details.

In germination experiments, t_{50} may be interpreted as the median germination time for the population of viable or non-dormant seeds only. This interpretation, however, depends on the assumption that all viable or non-dormant seeds have germinated by the end of the experiment, which may be established empirically by running the experiment until germination ceases and the maximum proportion becomes clearly discernible from the data.

In this chapter, we use the following extension packages:

```
library(drc)

library(devtools)
install_github("DoseResponse/drcData")
library(drcData)

library(lmtest)

library(metafor)

library(multcomp)

library(plyr)

library(sandwich)
```

5.1 Analysis of a single germination curve

5.1.1 Germination of *Stellaria media* seeds

We consider data from a germination test of chickweed (*Stellaria media*) seeds (Ritz *et al.*, 2013b). Seeds from a chlorsulfuron-resistant biotype were germinated in petri dishes (with a diameter of 9 cm) in a dark growth cabinet; we refer to Ritz *et al.* (2013b) for more details. The information about the petri dishes is no longer available. Two hundred seeds were placed on filter plates. At 34 consecutive inspection times, the number of germinated seeds was recorded and these seeds were removed. Definition of a germinated seed was the breakthrough of the seed testa by the radicle.

Data are available in the built-in dataset `chickweed` where there is one row per monitoring interval (in total 35 intervals when the interval after termination of the experiment is included). Note that the intervals need not have the same width and, furthermore, intervals without counts do not contribute to parameter estimation and could be left out. The first and last three lines of the dataset are shown below.

```
head(chickweed, 3)
```

```
##   start end count
## 1     0  12     0
## 2    12  22     0
## 3    22  30     0
```

```
tail(chickweed, 3)
```

```
##      start   end count
## 33 266.5 276.5     1
## 34 276.5 281.5     0
## 35 281.5   Inf   160
```

The columns named `start` and `end` contain the lower and upper limits of the monitoring intervals, whereas the column named `count` contains the number of seeds that germinated in the corresponding monitoring interval. The last row in the dataset contains the number of seeds that did not germinate during the experiment, with a monitoring interval ending at infinity (`Inf`).

Stellaria media has dormant seeds and therefore we would not expect 100% germination. Consequently, it is relevant to fit a three-parameter log-logistic model where the upper limit (the parameter d) corresponds to the total proportion germinated. The model is fitted using `drm()`, but the specification is slightly different from the one used in the previous chapters. The first argument in `drm()` is the model formula linking the response variable (`count`) on the left-hand side to the monitoring intervals, which are encoded by means of two variables (`start` and `end`) specified using + on the right-hand side of the formula. In addition, the argument `type` is equal to `"event"` to ensure that estimation is carried out by assuming the appropriate multinomial model as briefly explained above.

```
chickweed.LL.3 <- drm(count ~ start + end,
                      data = chickweed,
                      fct = LL.3(),
                      type = "event")
```

Before looking at the summary output, we make a residual plot to examine if the chosen model provides a reasonable description of the trend in the data. The residual plot in Figure 5.1 shows a clear curvilinear trend where residuals are first positive, then negative, then positive, and, finally, becoming negative again. This means the chosen model function is not providing a very good description of the trend in the data. It seems that there is much more nonlinearity in the data than captured by an s-shape. However, the residuals are small, in most cases being smaller than 0.01 (1% percentage point) and the detected departure will hardly be visible when we plot the fitted germination curve below, and it may not affect parameter estimates and standard errors much. It is also possible to construct a QQ plot as seen for continuous data

```
plot(fitted(chickweed.LL.3), residuals(chickweed.LL.3))
abline(h=0, lty=2)
qqnorm(residuals(chickweed.LL.3))
```

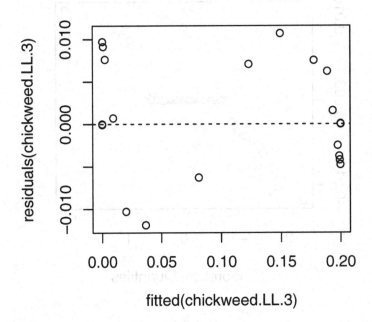

FIGURE 5.1
Residual plot for the three-parameter log-logistic model fitted to the dataset
chickweed.

but it should be kept in mind that the residuals will only be approximately
normally distributed and the many intervals without germination (if included)
will blur the picture somewhat (see Figure 5.2).

```
summary(chickweed.LL.3)

##
## Model fitted: Log-logistic (ED50 as parameter) with lower
##      limit at 0 (3 parms)
##
## Parameter estimates:
##
##                 Estimate Std. Error t-value   p-value
## b:(Intercept) -20.76732    2.94421 -7.0536 1.743e-12 ***
## d:(Intercept)   0.20011    0.02830  7.0711 1.537e-12 ***
## e:(Intercept) 196.05291    2.50572 78.2422 < 2.2e-16 ***
## ---
## Signif. codes: 0 '***' 0.001 '**' 0.01 '*' 0.05 '.' 0.1 ' ' 1
```

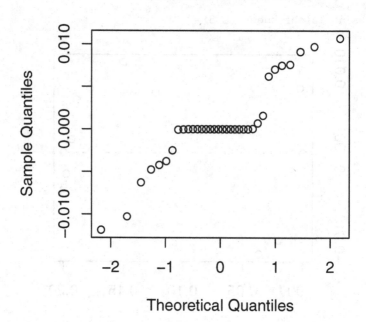

FIGURE 5.2
QQ plot of raw residuals from the three-parameter log-logistic model fitted to
the dataset `chickweed`.

The summary output reveals that only 20 (2.8) percent of the seeds germinated
during the experiment. Moreover, it took 196 (2.5) hours to germinate half of
the seeds that germinated during the experiment.

  One way to address this slight model misspecification caused by the cluster-
ing due to use of several petri dishes (even without having information about
which seeds belonged to which dish) is to use robust standard errors (see Section A.5 for more explanation). We need to activate the packages *lmtest* and
sandwich to be able to use the function `coeftest()` with the argument vcov.
= sandwich.

```
coeftest(chickweed.LL.3,
         vcov. = sandwich)
```

```
##
## t test of coefficients:
##
```

```
##                 Estimate Std. Error t value Pr(>|t|)
## b:(Intercept) -20.76732    7.84206 -2.6482  0.01246 *
## d:(Intercept)   0.20011    0.17438  1.1475  0.25967
## e:(Intercept) 196.05291    4.40685 44.4882  < 2e-16 ***
## ---
## Signif. codes: 0 '***' 0.001 '**' 0.01 '*' 0.05 '.' 0.1 ' ' 1
```

The resulting standard errors increased by a factor between 1.5 and 2.5, reflecting that the model was slightly misspecified.

Likewise, estimation of multiple time points corresponding to arbitrary percentages of germination with robust standard errors may be achieved using ED() with the same specification as in coeftest(). Below we estimate t_{10}, t_{50}, and t_{90} with robust standard errors and 95% confidence intervals.

```
ED(chickweed.LL.3,
   c(10, 50, 90),
   interval = "delta",
   vcov. = sandwich)
```

```
##
## Estimated effective doses
##
##           Estimate Std. Error   Lower     Upper
## e:1:10  176.3697      8.2987 160.1045 192.6349
## e:1:50  196.0529      4.4069 187.4156 204.6902
## e:1:90  217.9328      9.7192 198.8834 236.9821
```

It is also possible to estimate absolute germination times that refer to a total of 100% germination. As the estimated upper limit was just above 20% (0.20), it makes sense to estimate t_5, t_{10}, and t_{15}, the time it takes to reach 5%, 10%, and 15% germination of all seeds used. Again, we can use ED() but specifying proportions rather than percentages and using the argument type = "absolute" to switch from the default calculation relative to the estimated upper limit(s) to the absolute calculation. Which version is more relevant will depend on the application, but it should ideally be identified already during the planning phase of the experiment.

```
ED(chickweed.LL.3,
   c(0.05, 0.1, 0.15),
   interval = "delta",
   type = "absolute",
   vcov. = sandwich)
```

```
##
## Estimated effective doses
```

```
##
##          Estimate Std. Error   Lower    Upper
## e:1:0.05 185.9445     5.7647 174.6459 197.2431
## e:1:0.1  196.0425     4.4069 187.4053 204.6798
## e:1:0.15 206.6817     6.0136 194.8953 218.4680
```

Using the method `plot`, we show the fitted regression curve together with the cumulated proportions of germinated seeds. This plot may also serve as a kind of graphical model diagnostics. We add a confidence band based on 95% pointwise Wald-type confidence intervals, which may easily be obtained using the `predict()` method by providing a dataset of time points for which to obtain predicted values (in this case 0:300, corresponding to 0, 1, 2, ..., 300 hours). Figure 5.3 shows the resulting plot. The fitted germination curve seems to describe the increase in germination over time adequately.

As Wald-type confidence intervals are used for constructing the confidence band, the lower limit of the band would become slightly negative for around 180 hours if it were not truncated at 0. However, by default the `predict()` method has the argument `constrain` switched on so that truncation is enforced (whenever it is reasonable).

```
plot(chickweed.LL.3,
     xlim = c(0, 300), ylim = c(0, 0.30),
     xlab = "Time (hours)",
     ylab = "Proportion germinated",
     log = "")

chickweed.predicted <- predict(chickweed.LL.3,
                               data.frame(0:300),
                               interval = "confidence")

lines(0:300, chickweed.predicted[, "Lower"],
      col = "darkgray")

lines(0:300, chickweed.predicted[, "Upper"],
      col = "darkgray")
```

5.2   Analysis of data from multiple germination curves

It may often be relevant to compare germination among different groups or treatments. The corresponding experimental design will often lead to data for multiple germination curves, ideally per group or treatment. Had the response been continuous, a nonlinear mixed-effects dose-response model could possibly

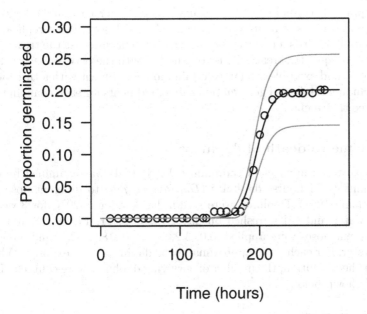

FIGURE 5.3
The germination curve based on the three-parameter log-logistic model fitted to the dataset `chickweed` plotted together with the observed cumulated proportions and a pointwise 95% confidence band.

have been fitted. To our knowledge no equivalent parametric random-effects models have been proposed for time-to-event data. A very flexible alternative is the two-step approach proposed by Jensen *et al.* (2017), extending the approach proposed by Jiang and Kopp-Schneider (2014) used in Subsection 1.2.2. We briefly outline the approach:

The first step consists of fitting a separate time-to-event-response model to data from each independent sub-experiment (e.g, batch, pot, or tray). From each model fit, estimates of parameters of interest (with corresponding estimated standard errors) are then collected in a new dataset. Information on all other variables related to the experimental design should also be gathered in the same dataset.

In the second step these estimates are used as response values for a meta analysis, which may be carried out by fitting a linear mixed model. In contrast to a usual linear mixed model, the residual standard error, which reflects variation within a sub-experiment, is not estimated. Instead, it is assumed to be known and equal to the estimated standard errors corresponding to the estimates. Inferential procedures such as pairwise comparisons based on approximate Wald-type u-tests are available, just like for an ordinary linear mixed model.

The approach is applied in two examples. In the first example, time-to-event-response curves were obtained for a number of doses without replication of germination. So it is a one-way layout without replication at the treatment level and, consequently, treatment is confounded with the between-curve variation. The second example is a large germination experiment with a three-way layout including replicated germination sub-experiments for each combination of the three treatments.

5.2.1   Time to death of daphnias

In a toxicity test the effect of cadmium chloride (Cd) was examined by exposing young (<24 hours) daphnias (*Daphnia magna*) to different doses of Cd (Kooijman, 1981). Daphnias were held in hard water at 20°C for 3 weeks with the water and Cd refreshed on day 2, 4, 7, 9, 11, 14, 16, 18 and 21. Seven different doses were applied: 0.0, 3.2, 5.6 10.0, 18.0, 32.0, and 56.0 μg Cd L^{-1} water. For each dose, approximately 50 daphnias were exposed. When refreshing the resolution, the number of surviving daphnias were counted. The dataset is shown below.

```
head(CadmiumDaphnia)
```

```
##    Dose Time Total Start End Dead
## 1  0.0    2    50     0   2    0
## 2  0.0    4    50     2   4    0
## 3  0.0    7    50     4   7    0
## 4  0.0    9    50     7   9    0
## 5  0.0   11    50     9  11    0
## 6  0.0   14    50    11  14    0
```

The dataset contains four variables: Dose denotes the dose of cadmium chloride, Start and End denote the limits on the monitoring intervals, and, finally, Dead denotes the number of dead daphnias recorded for the corresponding monitoring interval. Now we proceed to analyze these data using the meta-analytic approach.

5.2.1.1   Step 1

We will assume that a two-parameter log-logistic model will fit data for all doses. This may be highly questionable as all doses are not equally toxic. However, the duration of the experiment was not long enough to observe such differences. Moreover, it is not a limitation: different models for different doses is also possible as long as the same parameter of interest may be estimated.

We start out by manually fitting a two-parameter log-logistic model separately to data for each dose, and then estimated parameters from the resulting model fits are combined. It is a somewhat repetitive task, but it sheds some light on how the meta-analytic approach works. So we start out fitting 7 models, one per dose, using the function `subset()` for defining anonymous subsets on the fly.

```
daphnia.LL.2.00.0 <- drm(Dead ~ Start + End,
                         data = subset(CadmiumDaphnia, Dose == "0.0"),
                         fct = LL.2(),
                         type = "event")

daphnia.LL.2.03.2 <- drm(Dead ~ Start + End,
                         data = subset(CadmiumDaphnia, Dose == "3.2"),
                         fct = LL.2(),
                         type = "event")

daphnia.LL.2.05.6 <- drm(Dead ~ Start + End,
                         data = subset(CadmiumDaphnia, Dose == "5.6"),
                         fct = LL.2(),
                         type = "event")

daphnia.LL.2.10.0 <- drm(Dead ~ Start + End,
                         data = subset(CadmiumDaphnia, Dose == "10.0"),
                         fct = LL.2(),
                         type = "event")

daphnia.LL.2.18.0 <- drm(Dead ~ Start + End,
                         data = subset(CadmiumDaphnia, Dose == "18.0"),
                         fct = LL.2(),
                         type = "event")

daphnia.LL.2.32.0 <- drm(Dead ~ Start + End,
                         data = subset(CadmiumDaphnia, Dose == "32.0"),
                         fct = LL.2(),
                         type = "event")

daphnia.LL.2.56.0 <- drm(Dead ~ Start + End,
                         data = subset(CadmiumDaphnia, Dose == "56.0"),
                         fct = LL.2(),
                         type = "event")
```

The next step is to extract the estimated t_{50} and the corresponding standard error from each of the above model fits. For the two-parameter log-logistic model it is the estimate for the parameter e. We store the results in a dataset called `cadmium.t50`, which we initially define as an empty dataset.

```
cadmium.t50 <- data.frame(t50 = rep(NA, 7),
                          t50.se = rep(NA, 7))
```

Then the dataset is filled in row by row using `summary()` in combination with `coef()` for extracting estimates and standard errors.

```
cadmium.t50[1, ] <- coef(summary(daphnia.LL.2.00.0))[2, 1:2]

cadmium.t50[2, ] <- coef(summary(daphnia.LL.2.03.2))[2, 1:2]

cadmium.t50[3, ] <- coef(summary(daphnia.LL.2.05.6))[2, 1:2]

cadmium.t50[4, ] <- coef(summary(daphnia.LL.2.10.0))[2, 1:2]

cadmium.t50[5, ] <- coef(summary(daphnia.LL.2.18.0))[2, 1:2]

cadmium.t50[6, ] <- coef(summary(daphnia.LL.2.32.0))[2, 1:2]

cadmium.t50[7, ] <- coef(summary(daphnia.LL.2.56.0))[2, 1:2]
```

The manual fitting of 7 models could have been avoided using a call of `drm()`
with the argument `curveid` to assume different model parameters for different
doses. The R lines are shown below but are not executed; we invite the reader
to do so.

```
daphnia.LL.2 <- drm(Dead ~ Start + End,
                curveid = as.factor(Dose),
                data = CadmiumDaphnia,
                fct = LL.2(),
                type = "event")
```

```
cadmium.t50x <- coef(summary(daphnia.LL.2))[8:14, 1:2]
colnames(cadmium.t50x) <- c("t50", "t50.se")
```

In theory, exactly the same parameter estimates and standard errors could
then be obtained in one go. However, in practice, parameter estimates and
standard errors may be slightly different as fitting this model involves estimation of $7 + 7 = 14$ parameter simultaneously. In general, it is more challenging
to fit such simultaneous models as lack of convergence and convergence to sub-
optimal parameter estimates may often occur, i.e., the estimation procedure
may have problems in case many parameters need to be estimated. Assuming
a shared parameter across doses (a shared slope parameter b) would be an
option (by means of the argument `pmodels` used in the same way as previously in Subsection 1.2.1). However, we believe it will in practice be difficult
to justify such assumptions based on a priori knowledge about the underlying biological mechanisms. Moreover, as you will see in the next example (in
Subsection 5.2.2), fitting separate models to subsets of a dataset may be automated since it better scales up for more complex experimental designs, also
when it comes to merging relevant information about the experimental design
with the estimates obtained. To ensure that all relevant information is carried

over to the second step, we add a column to the dataset with information on the doses.

```
cadmium.t50 <- data.frame(Dose = c(0, 3.2, 5.6, 10, 18, 32, 56),
                          cadmium.t50)

cadmium.t50

##   Dose       t50      t50.se
## 1  0.0 23.412632   6.3833146
## 2  3.2 74.466687  69.9816272
## 3  5.6 38.331515  10.3035074
## 4 10.0 35.720487   8.2251577
## 5 18.0 11.034994   1.0383054
## 6 32.0  5.192387   0.3324163
## 7 56.0  1.954142   0.1575264
```

The scatterplot in Figure 5.4 shows the estimated t_{50} values as a function of dose. A distinct nonlinear trend is discernible but the variation in the estimates time-to-event seems to depend on the magnitude of the estimates: the larger the estimate, the larger the variation.

5.2.1.2   Step 2

We use the package *metafor* to combine estimates from the individual model fits into pooled estimates through the meta-analytic approach (Viechtbauer, 2010). Specifically we use the function rma(), which takes the estimated t_{50} as the first argument and the corresponding *squared* standard errors as the second argument. The explanatory variables are specified through a formula in the argument mods. Finally, the argument data is used for providing the dataset where the variables given in the first three arguments are found. Specifically, we fit a weighted version of a linear regression model for the logarithm-transformed t_{50} as a function of dose through the specification mods =   Dose, exploiting that the estimated standard error for a logarithm-transformed estimate is the estimated standard error of the untransformed variable divided by the estimate itself (which may be obtained using the delta method). The reason for applying a logarithm transformation is that the summary output showing increased variation with increased estimated t_{50} values and, at the same time, this transformation may remedy some of the observed nonlinearity seen in the below plot (Figure 5.4).

```
cadmium.t50.log.oneway <- rma(log(t50),
                              (t50.se/t50)^2,
                              mods= ~ Dose,
                              data = cadmium.t50)
```

```
plot(t50 ~ Dose,
     data = cadmium.t50,
     xlab = "Dose (mu g Cd/L)",
     ylab = "Time to 50% died")
```

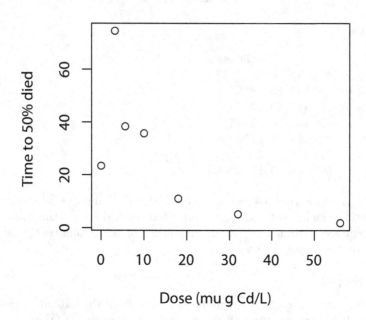

FIGURE 5.4
Estimated t_{50} values from the first step in the meta-analytic approach as a function of dose of cadmium chloride (using the dataset `CadmiumDaphnia`).

`coef()` applied to the summary output provides a condensed version of the summary output, only containing information on the parameter estimates for the linear regression.

```
coef(summary(cadmium.t50.log.oneway))
```

```
##            estimate          se       zval         pval       ci.lb
## intrcpt  3.63528901 0.234205039 15.521822 2.469372e-54  3.17625557
## Dose    -0.05508716 0.007800124 -7.062344 1.637174e-12 -0.07037512
##             ci.ub
## intrcpt  4.0943225
## Dose    -0.0397992
```

The logarithm-transformed t_{50} decreases significantly with increasing dose ($p < 0.0001$): for each increase in the dose of 1 μg Cd L^{-1} the average t_{50} value is reduced by 5.4 percent (we can claim a relative reduction as consequence of using a logarithm transformation). It is worth mentioning that the meta-analytic approach on untransformed estimated t_{50} values (assuming a linear trend in dose) showed no significant effect of dose.

The `predict()` method in *metafor* can be used to obtain predicted values for the fitted regression line along with the corresponding (pointwise) confidence intervals. The argument `newmods` is used for specifying the doses for which a prediction is needed. We ask for predicted values for doses between 0 and 60 at increments of 1.

```
cadmium.predicted <- predict(cadmium.t50.log.oneway,
                             newmods = seq(0, 60, by = 1))

head(cadmium.predicted)

##      pred     se ci.lb ci.ub  cr.lb  cr.ub
## 1 3.6353 0.2342 3.1763 4.0943 2.8436 4.4270
## 2 3.5802 0.2283 3.1328 4.0276 2.7952 4.3652
## 3 3.5251 0.2225 3.0891 3.9611 2.7466 4.3037
## 4 3.4700 0.2168 3.0452 3.8949 2.6977 4.2424
## 5 3.4149 0.2112 3.0010 3.8289 2.6485 4.1814
## 6 3.3599 0.2058 2.9565 3.7632 2.5991 4.1206
```

The predicted values are found in the first column named `pred`, whereas the third and fourth columns contain the lower and upper limits of the (95%) confidence intervals (named `ci.lb` and `ci.ub`, respectively). Note that predicted values and confidence intervals are back-transformed from the logarithmic scale to the original time scale using the exponential function `exp()`.

So we can redraw the scatterplot with the fitted nonlinear curve and confidence band (Figure 5.5). The fitted regression curve describes the average trend in the data quite satisfactorily.

5.2.2 A hierarchical three-way factorial design

We consider data from a greenhouse trial studying seedling emergence for an herbicide-susceptible (S) and an herbicide-resistant (R) blackgrass sub-population, both isolated from a single population (Keshtkar *et al.*, 2017). For two different temperature regimes, seedling emergence in the two sub-populations was investigated under four different sowing depths. For each of the 16 combinations of depth, sub-population, and temperature, four pots with 36 seeds were used and germination was monitored for 22–43 days at intervals of varying lengths for the two temperatures (21–22 monitoring intervals). The pots were arranged in a completely randomized design with four repetitions of each combination of the three factors. This completely randomized experiment was conducted twice. Thus, the experimental design was a completely randomized three-way factorial layout with 2 blocks. We refer to Keshtkar *et al.* (2017) for more information on the experiment.

```
plot(t50 ~ Dose,
     data = cadmium.t50,
     xlab = "Dose (mu g Cd/L)",
     ylab = "Time to 50% died")

lines(0:60,
      exp(cadmium.predicted[["pred"]]), lty = 1)   # fitted line

lines(0:60,
      exp(cadmium.predicted[["ci.lb"]]), lty = 2)   # lower CI

lines(0:60,
      exp(cadmium.predicted[["ci.ub"]]), lty = 2)   # upper CI
```

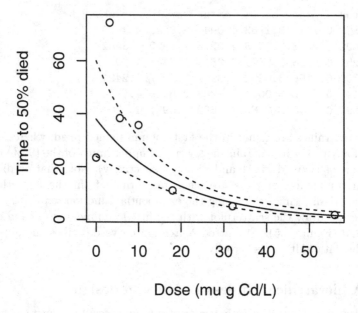

FIGURE 5.5
Estimated t_{50} values from the first step in the meta-analytic approach plotted vs. doses of cadmium chloride (using the dataset `CadmiumDaphnia`). The fitted and back-transformed regression curve (solid line) with a 95% confidence band (dashed lines) is also shown.

Data are in the dataset `blackgrass`. The three treatments are encoded in the variables `Bio`, `Depth`, and `Temp`.

```
head(blackgrass)
```

```
##   Exp Temp Popu Bio Depth Rep Start.Day End.Day Ger Accum.Ger TotalSeed
## 1   1   10  914   S     0   1         0     360   0         0        36
```

```
## 2   1   10   914   S      0   1        360      376   0            0         36
## 3   1   10   914   S      0   1        376      384   0            0         36
## 4   1   10   914   S      0   1        384      400   0            0         36
## 5   1   10   914   S      0   1        400      408   0            0         36
## 6   1   10   914   S      0   1        408      424   0            0         36
```

For the first experiment, the data may be tabulated as follows.

```
with(subset(blackgrass, Exp == 1), table(Depth, Bio, Temp))
```

```
## , , Temp = 10
##
##       Bio
## Depth  R  S
##     0 88 88
##     1 88 88
##     3 88 88
##     6 88 88
##
## , , Temp = 17
##
##       Bio
## Depth  R  S
##     0 84 84

##     1 84 84
##     3 84 84
##     6 84 84
```

The numbers 88 and 84 correspond to 22 or 21 monitoring intervals in four replicates (pots), respectively.

The experimental design is encoded through the variables Exp and Rep, where the latter is the identifier variable for pots in the dataset. It is, however, not unique as multiple instances of Rep equal to 1 occur (in different sub-experiments) as seen from the following table.

```
with(blackgrass, table (Exp, Rep))
```

```
##     Rep
## Exp   1    2    3    4
##   1 344  344  344  344
##   2 344  344  344  344
```

Therefore, we start out adding such a variable (given the name Pot) to the dataset blackgrass. It would be nice if such a unique identifier were always included in such datasets as it may help understand where the random variation in the data is introduced.

```
blackgrass[["Pot"]] <- with(blackgrass,
                    as.numeric(interaction(Exp, Bio, Depth,
                                            Temp, Rep)))
```

Pot has 128 levels, corresponding to a total of 128 pots being used in the experiment. Now we are ready to begin analyzing the data using the two-step approach.

5.2.2.1   Step 1

A three-parameter log-logistic model is fitted to data from each pot separately. We show how to do this in an automated way, avoiding fitting a model manually for each pot.

Looping through data from all pots and fitting a dose-response model to data from each pot separately may effectively be carried out using the **R** package *plyr* in combination with the following helper function that defines what has to be done for each pot (in this case fitting an LL.3() model). Note that if you need to use different model functions within the same experiment (e.g., both LL.2() and LL.3()) then automation may become more difficult as a systematic approach for model selection is needed. In the code below dataSet is a placeholder for the subset provided to the function applied for each pot.

```
fitFct.LL.3 <- function(dataSet)
{
    modelFit <- try(drm(Ger ~ Start.Day + End.Day,
                    data = dataSet,
                    fct = LL.3(),
                    type = "event"), silent = TRUE)

    if (inherits(modelFit, "try-error")) {modelFit <- NULL}

    return(modelFit)
}
```

The model may not converge for all pots, which is the reason why we use try() inside the helper function; this function will catch all errors and, thereby, ensure that fitting a lot of models in a loop, as shown below, will not terminate prematurely due to a few cases with lack of convergence and resulting in no model fits. For germination data, lack of convergence can happen because of a low number of seedlings emerging or because all emerging seedlings emerge at the same or at very few times. In both cases, it may be difficult to fit any dose-response model. Sometimes manual fitting for problematic cases may still result in a useful model fit being obtained, but it is more cumbersome and, if different model functions are assumed, results may be not be fully comparable between automatic and manual model fits.

We use the function dlply() from *plyr* for the actual looping: For data corresponding to each combination of the three treatment variables Bio, Depth, and Temp and the grouping variables Exp and Pot, reflecting the hierarchical design, the above-defined function fitFct.LL.3() is applied. Note that combining these 5 variables yield many more combinations than actually present in the dataset, but it ensures that the experimental design is carried along with the estimates. dlply() takes a dataset (data frame) as input and returns a list.

```
black.grass.modelfits2 <- dlply(blackgrass,
                      .(Exp, Bio, Depth, Temp, Pot),
                      fitFct.LL.3)
```

The list black.grass.modelfits2 is quite large and you may not want to look at it as it is. We proceed to extract the three parameter estimates and corresponding estimated standard errors from each model fit. For that purpose, we use another helper function as defined below.

```
paramFct.LL.3 <- function(fitObj)
{
  if (is.null(fitObj)) {return(rep(NA, 6))}
  # handling replicates with all values missing

  coefSum <- coef(summary(fitObj))
  returnVec <- c(coefSum[1, 1:2],   # slope
              coefSum[2, 1:2],   # maximum
              ED(fitObj, 50, display = FALSE)[1:2])   # t50

  names(returnVec) <- c("b", "b.se",
                    "d", "d.se",
                    "t50", "t50.se")
  # adding column names

  returnVec
}
```

Again, we exploit functionality from the extension package *plyr* for looping through the list of model fits (black.grass.modelfits2). This time we use the function ldply(), which takes a list and returns a dataset. Note also that we estimate t_{50} values that are relative to the estimated upper limits (this could be changed using the argument type = "absolute" as seen previously in Subsection 5.2.1).

```
blackgrass.parms <- ldply(black.grass.modelfits2, paramFct.LL.3)
```

```
summary(blackgrass.parms)
```

```
##       Exp      Bio      Depth          Temp            Pot
## Min.   :1.0  R:64  Min.   :0.00  Min.   :10.0  Min.   :  1.00
## 1st Qu.:1.0  S:64  1st Qu.:0.75  1st Qu.:10.0  1st Qu.: 32.75
## Median :1.5        Median :2.00  Median :13.5  Median : 64.50
## Mean   :1.5        Mean   :2.50  Mean   :13.5  Mean   : 64.50
## 3rd Qu.:2.0        3rd Qu.:3.75  3rd Qu.:17.0  3rd Qu.: 96.25
## Max.   :2.0        Max.   :6.00  Max.   :17.0  Max.   :128.00
##
##       b                    b.se                d
## Min.   :-321.593    Min.   :  0.4799   Min.   :-1041.3839
## 1st Qu.: -13.253    1st Qu.:  1.6114   1st Qu.:    0.4171
## Median : -10.042    Median :  2.1744   Median :    0.6113
## Mean   : -22.468    Mean   : 34.8117   Mean   :   -7.9552
## 3rd Qu.:  -8.183    3rd Qu.:  2.7119   3rd Qu.:    0.7780
## Max.   :   2.735    Max.   :847.1601   Max.   :    1.7379
## NA's   :6           NA's   :6          NA's   :6
##       d.se                t50            t50.se
## Min.   :  0.02737   Min.   :201.5   Min.   :  1.764
## 1st Qu.:  0.06949   1st Qu.:241.0   1st Qu.:  7.269
## Median :  0.07857   Median :440.7   Median : 17.958
## Mean   :  1.52145   Mean   :429.8   Mean   : 28.087
##
## 3rd Qu.:  0.08271   3rd Qu.:549.2   3rd Qu.: 26.911
## Max.   :173.79139   Max.   :823.2   Max.   :528.089
## NA's   :6           NA's   :6       NA's   :6
```

From the summary of the resulting dataset named `blackgrass.parms` we see
that there are 6 missing values (NAs) in the dataset. Therefore, for some pots
the three-parameter log-logistic model could not be fitted.

5.2.2.2   Step 2

The second step of the analysis is fitting the meta-analytic random-effects
model for the parameter(s) of interest. We only consider a model for $t50$.
However, the same approach could be applied to the analysis of the slope and
maximum germination parameters.

Specifically, we consider a model that can be formulated as follows.

$$\text{Estimated } t_{50,i} = \mu(\text{Temperature}_i, \text{Bio}_i, \text{Depth}_i) + A(\text{experiment}_i) + \theta_i + \varepsilon_i,$$

where i refers to the independent sampling units in the experiment, the μ
values denote the parameters signifying the mean t_{50} levels for the treatment
combinations of the interaction; A is a random effect capturing differences

between experiments; θ is the random effect explaining the heterogeneity between pots (nested within experiment); and ε is the residual error. Random effects and residual errors are assumed to be mutually independent and normally distributed with mean 0. The standard deviations of the random effects are unknown and have to be estimated from data and the standard deviations of the residual errors are assumed to be known and equal to the estimated standard errors of the estimates. Hence, the smaller the standard error in a pot-specific analysis in Step 1, the larger the weight of the corresponding estimate in the meta-analytic model fit in Step 2.

To estimate the average time to 50% emergence for each combination of the three treatments, a new variable that corresponds to the three-way interaction of `Bio`, `Depth`, and `Temp` is added to the dataset. Introducing such a variable will allow us to define relevant pairwise comparisons, which is much more interesting than testing interactions in the three-way factorial layout.

```
blackgrass.parms[["BioDepthTemp"]] <-
  with(blackgrass.parms, interaction(Bio, Depth, Temp))
```

We use the function `rma.mv()` in the package *metafor* (Viechtbauer, 2010) for estimating the random-effects meta-analytic model. The default method for estimation is REML.

```
blackgrass.t50.mm <- rma.mv(t50, (t50.se)^2,
                  mods= ~ BioDepthTemp - 1,
                  random= ~ 1|Exp/Pot,
                  data = blackgrass.parms)
```

```
## Warning in rma.mv(t50, (t50.se)^2, mods = ~BioDepthTemp - 1,
random = ~1 | : Rows with NAs omitted from model fitting.
```

The specification `Exp/Pot` ensures that the hierarchical structure of the experimental design is also incorporated in the statistical analysis. A warning message is issued because missing values occurred and were left out of the analysis. It reflects that for some pots the three-parameter log-logistic model could not be fitted. However, as pointed out previously, it may still be possible to fit models for these pots manually.

To obtain a condensed summary output with estimates, standard errors, and confidence intervals, the `coef()` method may be used.

```
coef(summary(blackgrass.t50.mm))[, c("estimate", "se",
                                "ci.lb", "ci.ub")]
```

```
##                    estimate       se    ci.lb    ci.ub
## BioDepthTempR.0.10 684.3207 11.769466 661.2529 707.3884
## BioDepthTempS.0.10 656.2772 11.674943 633.3947 679.1596
```

```
## BioDepthTempR.1.10 503.2574 12.036954 479.6654 526.8494
## BioDepthTempS.1.10 478.0808 10.285295 457.9220 498.2396
## BioDepthTempR.3.10 521.1635 10.938573 499.7243 542.6027
## BioDepthTempS.3.10 464.3360  9.918119 444.8968 483.7751
## BioDepthTempR.6.10 605.4620 21.880176 562.5776 648.3463
## BioDepthTempS.6.10 579.8046 11.720794 556.8322 602.7769
## BioDepthTempR.0.17 374.9668 11.346542 352.7279 397.2056
## BioDepthTempS.0.17 375.9767 10.723558 354.9590 396.9945
## BioDepthTempR.1.17 227.7426  8.527922 211.0281 244.4570
## BioDepthTempS.1.17 213.1403  8.024740 197.4121 228.8685
## BioDepthTempR.3.17 227.5065  8.058943 211.7112 243.3017
## BioDepthTempS.3.17 211.6396  7.969696 196.0193 227.2599
## BioDepthTempR.6.17 296.5767 11.850070 273.3510 319.8024
## BioDepthTempS.6.17 261.9117  9.510475 243.2716 280.5519
```

The summary output (see below) also contains the estimated standard deviations for the experiment and pot-specific random effects. These estimates would be useful to report in a publication to give some insight in how random variation is split into between-experiment and between-pot variation (we observe that the standard deviation describing the between-pot variation is approximately a factor 3 larger than the standard deviation describing the between-experiment variation).

```
summary(blackgrass.t50.mm)[["sigma2"]]
```

```
## [1]   44.10246 305.80208
```

All pairwise comparisons may conveniently be defined using the following contrast matrix:

```
allPairWiseComp <- contrMat(coef(blackgrass.t50.mm), "Tukey")
```

All pairwise comparisons with unadjusted p-values are then calculated (but not shown) using glht().

```
blackgrass.allpairwise <- glht(blackgrass.t50.mm,
                       linfct = allPairWiseComp)
```

To have all comparisons shown, the summary() method may be used.

```
summary(blackgrass.allpairwise,
        test = adjusted(type = "none"))
```

We do not show the output as it would contain numerous pairwise comparisons, of which only a few may be relevant. Note that multiplicity adjustment of p-values was switched off manually (using test = adjusted(type =

"none") as adjustment is applied by default). It is much better to ask for certain relevant comparisons. Among other things, Keshtkar *et al.* (2017) looked at comparisons between sub-populations for each depth and each temperature. To obtain the relevant comparisons we define a targeted contrast matrix.

```
targetedPairWiseComp <-
  c("BioDepthTempR.0.10 - BioDepthTempS.0.10 = 0",
    "BioDepthTempR.1.10 - BioDepthTempS.1.10 = 0",
    "BioDepthTempR.3.10 - BioDepthTempS.3.10 = 0",
    "BioDepthTempR.6.10 - BioDepthTempS.6.10 = 0",
    "BioDepthTempR.0.17 - BioDepthTempS.0.17 = 0",
    "BioDepthTempR.1.17 - BioDepthTempS.1.17 = 0",
    "BioDepthTempR.3.17 - BioDepthTempS.3.17 = 0",
    "BioDepthTempR.6.17 - BioDepthTempS.6.17 = 0")
```

The names of combinations as found in the summary output of the model fit should be used. It is also important to include -1 in the model specification as otherwise the parameterization will not allow the above specification of contrasts. We can use glht() and the corresponding summary() method to show the comparisons.

```
blackgrass.targeted.pairwise <- glht(blackgrass.t50.mm,
                       linfct = targetedPairWiseComp)

summary(blackgrass.targeted.pairwise)

##
##    Simultaneous Tests for General Linear Hypotheses
##
## Fit: rma.mv(yi = t50, V = (t50.se)^2, mods = ~BioDepthTemp - 1,
##      random = ~1 | Exp/Pot, data = blackgrass.parms)
##
## Linear Hypotheses:
##                                          Estimate Std. Error z value
## BioDepthTempR.0.10 - BioDepthTempS.0.10 == 0    28.043      15.186   1.847
## BioDepthTempR.1.10 - BioDepthTempS.1.10 == 0    25.177      14.372   1.752
## BioDepthTempR.3.10 - BioDepthTempS.3.10 == 0    56.828      13.189   4.309
## BioDepthTempR.6.10 - BioDepthTempS.6.10 == 0    25.657      23.846   1.076
## BioDepthTempR.0.17 - BioDepthTempS.0.17 == 0    -1.010      14.119  -0.072
## BioDepthTempR.1.17 - BioDepthTempS.1.17 == 0    14.602       9.644   1.514
## BioDepthTempR.3.17 - BioDepthTempS.3.17 == 0    15.867       9.185   1.728
## BioDepthTempR.6.17 - BioDepthTempS.6.17 == 0    34.665      13.697   2.531
##                                          Pr(>|z|)
## BioDepthTempR.0.10 - BioDepthTempS.0.10 == 0 0.414905
## BioDepthTempR.1.10 - BioDepthTempS.1.10 == 0 0.485949
## BioDepthTempR.3.10 - BioDepthTempS.3.10 == 0 0.000131 ***
## BioDepthTempR.6.10 - BioDepthTempS.6.10 == 0 0.929323
## BioDepthTempR.0.17 - BioDepthTempS.0.17 == 0 1.000000
## BioDepthTempR.1.17 - BioDepthTempS.1.17 == 0 0.671768
```

```
## BioDepthTempR.3.17 - BioDepthTempS.3.17 == 0 0.504652
## BioDepthTempR.6.17 - BioDepthTempS.6.17 == 0 0.087475 .
## ---
## Signif. codes: 0 '***' 0.001 '**' 0.01 '*' 0.05 '.' 0.1 ' ' 1
## (Adjusted p values reported -- single-step method)
```

We only find a significant difference between resistant and susceptible sub-populations for depth 3 cm and the 10/5°C temperature regime: in the resistant sub-population seedlings emerged 57 (13) hours later.

6

Benchmark dose estimation

Benchmark doses are in a sense parallel to the concept of effective doses (see Section A.13) (Ritz *et al.*, 2013a), but while the latter usually occurs in a dose-region with a reasonable amount of data available, the benchmark dose estimation is essentially an interpolation method for the low-dose region where little or no data is present.

To define a benchmark dose (BMD) we first need to define the background level, p_0, as the probability of an adverse response for an unexposed population. This level could be taken from the literature, estimated from data, or pre-specified at a fixed level such as 0.05. A benchmark response or benchmark risk (BMR) is a small increase above the background level in the probability of an adverse event. The BMD is the dose eliciting a response equal to BMR on average, assuming some dose-response model.

Usually risk assessment is not based on the BMD itself but on the benchmark dose lower limit (BMDL), which is defined as the lower limit of the confidence interval for the BMD (Crump, 1984). As the estimate of BMDL is partly determined by the uncertainty of the BMD estimate, it penalizes poor designs and analysis strategies.

The BMDL may be found using different approaches. The simplest approach proposed by Crump (Crump, 1984) is using a one-sided Wald-type confidence interval. However, it may result in negative BMDLs. One simple solution may be to combine the Wald-type confidence intervals with a transformation (typically the logarithm) to avoid negative values (Buckley *et al.*, 2009; Namata *et al.*, 2008; Moon *et al.*, 2013). Other approaches for estimating the BMDL include finding the dose associated with the upper limit of the confidence band of the fitted dose-response curve (inverse regression) (Buckley *et al.*, 2009; Fang *et al.*, 2015), different bootstrap strategies (Buckley *et al.*, 2009; Piegorsch *et al.*, 2012, 2014; Zhu *et al.*, 2007) and profile likelihood intervals (Yu and Catalano, 2005; Izadi *et al.*, 2012; Fox *et al.*, 2017; Ringblom *et al.*, 2014).

In this chapter, we use the following extension packages:

```
library(drc)
```

```
library(devtools)
install_github("DoseResponse/drcData")
library(drcData)
```

```
install_github("DoseResponse/bmd")
library(bmd)

library(metafor)

library(sandwich)
```

6.1 Binomial dose-response data

For all binomial responses, BMD may be defined in the same way as data share a common response scale (Crump, 1984). Two common definitions are used: Added or additional risk:

$$BMR = f(BMD, \beta) - p_0 \tag{6.1}$$

Excess or extra risk:

$$BMR = \frac{f(BMD, \beta) - p_0}{1 - p_0} \tag{6.2}$$

The excess risk definition is recommended by several authorities (U. S. EPA, 2012; Hardy *et al.*, 2017). When the background risk is 0 the two definitions are identical and thus result in the same BMD.

6.1.1 Pathogens in food

A total of 108 healthy human volunteers participated in a study of the effect of different doses of the pathogen, *Echovirus 12*. Each participant was exposed to the pathogen in one of four doses. Based on measurement of blood samples, it was determined whether or not the exposure had led to an infection. Data were reported by Moon *et al.* (2013). The full dataset is shown below. The dose of the pathogen is reported in plague forming units (pfu).

```
head(echovirus)
```

```
##    dose total infected
## 1   330    50       15
## 2  1000    20        9
## 3  3300    26       19
## 4 10000    12       12
```

As seen from the data, more people were exposed to the lower doses than to the higher. This has two major advantages: Fewer people will experience an adverse effect and we get more information about the low dose area, which we are interested in when considering benchmark doses.

The purpose of this study was to estimate the BMD_{10}, i.e., to find the safe dose associated with a predefined acceptable level, BMR = 10% increase over the background level, of pathogen-specific infections. For the dataset *echovirus*, this involves extrapolation, which we would usually recommend to avoid. However, in the present case one could argue that we also know that no one will be infected unless they are exposed to the specific pathogen. This means we have the extra information that a potential dose 0 would result in no infections. In practice, this information is incorporated in our model fitting by assuming the background level is 0. Accordingly, we fit a two-parameter log-logistic model.

```
pathogen.m1 <- drm(infected/total ~ dose,
                   weights = total,
                   data = echovirus,
                   fct = LL.2(),
                   type = "binomial")
```

In this case, we are interested in finding the dose that results in 10% being infected. Figure 6.1 shows the data together with the estimated dose-response model (**R** lines for the plot are provided in Subsection C.2.1). The figure illustrates how BMD can be found as the dose resulting in the level of risk determined by the pre-specified level of BMR.

We use the package *bmd* to estimate the BMD and the corresponding BMDL as follows:

```
bmd(pathogen.m1,
    0.10,
    def = "additional",
    backgType = "modelBased")

##        BMD      BMDL
##   90.32084  10.0272
```

The estimated BMD resulting in 10% being infected is 90.3 pfu with a BMDL of 10.0 pfu based on a Wald-type confidence interval that relies on asymptotic, large-sample results on the behaviour of parameter estimates.

The default method for finding BMDL in `bmd()` is using the lower limit of Wald-type confidence intervals. An alternative approach for estimating BMDL is to use a bootstrap method, which does not, to the same degree, depend on asymptotic results. We choose a parametric bootstrap approach where new datasets are generated from a binomial distribution with parameters $(N_i, N_i/Y_i)$ for each dose, i, separately. Here N_i refers to the total number in dose group i and Y_i refers to the number of infected in dose group i. The

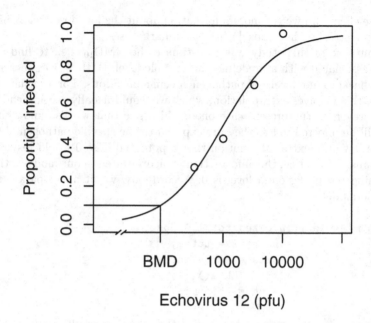

FIGURE 6.1
Two-parameter log-logistic model fitted to the dataset *echovirus*. With a background level of 0, BMD is the dose associated with the risk equal to the pre-specified BMR of 0.10.

BMDL is defined as the 5% percentile in the bootstrap distribution of BMDs (using the percentile interval).

```
pathogen.bmd.boot <- bmdBoot(pathogen.m1,
                    0.10,
                    def = "additional",
                    backgType = "modelBased",
                    bootType = "parametric",
                    R = 1000,
                    display = FALSE)
pathogen.bmd.boot$Result
```

```
##        BMD      BMDL
## 90.32084 28.78989
```

The BMDL found by the bootstrap method is much higher than the BMDL we found above. It may be caused by the relatively few doses in the present study and the fact that we work with binomial data. A simple histogram of bootstrap estimates (Figure 6.2) shows that the distribution is skewed and

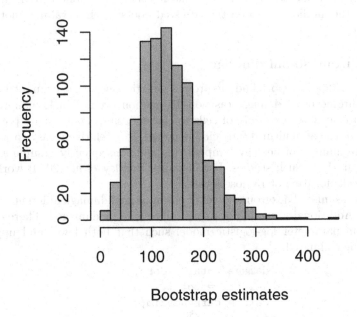

FIGURE 6.2
Histogram of the distribution of the bootstrap estimates used for estimating BMDL for the dataset *echovirus*.

further investigations will reveal a dependence between the estimate and the bootstrap standard error. This phenomenon is well known when working with distributions like the binomial where the variance is a function of the mean (Hesterberg, 2015). Consequently, using the percentile bootstrap confidence interval can give misleading estimates of the BMDL.

As an alternative to the default percentile interval, the function *bmdBoot()* has an option called "BCa" for the argument `bootInterval` using a bias-corrected and adjusted bootstrap interval (DiCiccio and Efron, 1996).

```
bmdBoot(pathogen.m1,
        0.10,
        def = "additional",
        backgType = "modelBased",
        bootType = "parametric",
        R = 1000,
        bootInterval = "BCa")

##        BMD       BMDL
## 90.32084 27.51616
```

The corrected bootstrap interval results in almost the same BMDL, indicating that the method based on the adjusted bootstrap interval may not be needed here.

6.1.2   Chromosomal damage

Bentley *et al.* (2000) report findings from a genetic study that examined the potential chromosomal damage (as non-disjunction events) in human lymphocytes after in vitro exposure of cells to carbendazim, a potentially potent metabolite of the agricultural fungicide benomyl. It is relatively easy to work with a large number of healthy lymphocytes and consequently, sample sizes can grow quickly in such studies. For instance, Bentley *et al.* (2000) worked with 2000 cells for each of 13 dose levels.

We will assume a background level of chromosomal damage different from 0, above 0. Additionally, we do not expect all cells to be damaged. Therefore, we fit a four-parameter log-logistic model such that both lower and upper limits will be estimated.

```
carbendazim.m1 <- drm(damage/total ~ dose,
                      weights = total,
                      data = carbendazim,
                      fct = LL.4(),
                      type = "binomial")
```

There are only data in the low dose region, i.e., the region of doses leading to small effects (Figure 6.3). Therefore it is possible to look at small BMRs. For this example, we will consider BMR = 0.01. The background risk is estimated by the model to be 0.00825. Assuming additional risk, the BMD is the dose resulting in a proportion of damaged cells equal to 0.00825 + 0.01 = 0.01825.

```
bmd(carbendazim.m1,
    0.01,
    def = "additional",
    backgType = "modelBased")
```

```
##      BMD      BMDL
## 756.442 683.1871
```

Alternatively, we could consider the excess risk definition. Still using the estimated background level, BMD is the dose associated with a proportion of cells being damaged of 0.01816 (0.01·(1-0.00825)+0.00825).

```
bmd(carbendazim.m1,
    0.01,
    def = "excess",
    backgType = "modelBased")
```

```
##       BMD      BMDL
## 754.9196 682.057
```

```
plot(carbendazim.m1,
    broken = TRUE,
    xlab = "Carbendazim (ng/ml)",
    ylab = "Proportion of damaged cells")
```

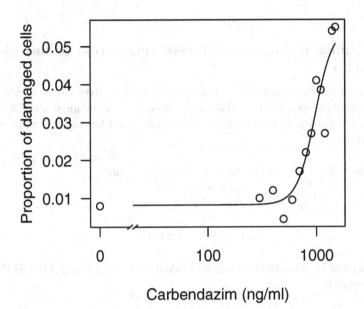

FIGURE 6.3
Four-parameter log-logistic model fitted to the dataset `carbendazim`.

For this example with a low background risk, the difference between additional and excess is small. Looking at the definition of BMD in (6.1) and (6.2) this is not surprising. For $p_0 \approx 0$ they both reduce to $BMR = f(BMD, \beta)$.

Finally, if we knew from the literature that the background level is actually 0.01, then the BMD associated with a BMR = 0.01 is found by specifying a user-defined background level, which will overrule any estimated background level. The BMD is then the dose associated with a proportion of cells being damaged equal to 0.0199 (0.01·(1-0.01)+0.01).

```
bmd(carbendazim.m1,
    0.01,
    def = "excess",
```

```
        backgType = "absolute",
        backg = 0.01)

##         BMD        BMDL
## 785.8377 703.7944
```

6.1.3   Tumor incidence continued: Integration of historical data

We return to the data from Subsection 2.1.2 describing liver tumor incidence in female Sprague-Dawley rats that were exposed to a chemical like 2,3,7,8-tetrachlorodibenzo-p-dioxin (TCDD). A two-parameter log-logistic model was fitted to data.

```
liver.tumor.LL.2 <- drm(incidence/total ~ conc,
                        weights = total,
                        data = liver.tumor,
                        fct = LL.2(),
                        type = "binomial")
```

Finding the BMD corresponding to a BMR = 0.1 using excess risk is then straightforward.

```
BMD.NTP <- bmd(liver.tumor.LL.2,
               0.1,
               def = "excess",
               backgType = "modelBased",
               display = FALSE)

BMD.NTP$Results

##        BMD      BMDL
## 23.90412 20.651
```

The data are from a National Toxicology Program (NTP) study (National Toxicology Program, 2006). Other studies, however, examined the same endpoints using the same species, sex, and exposure method. For instance, the dataset below is from a similar study examining the effect of TCDD on liver tumors in female Sprague-Dawley rats (Kociba *et al.*, 1978).

```
head(TCDD)
```

```
##    conc total incidence
## 1  0.00    86         2
## 2  1.55    50         1
## 3  7.15    50         9
## 4 38.56    45        14
```

```
liver.tumor.Kociba.LL.2 <- drm(incidence/total ~ conc,
                               weights = total,
                               data = TCDD,
                               fct = LL.2(),
                               type = "binomial")
```

```
BMD.Kociba <- bmd(liver.tumor.Kociba.LL.2,
                  0.1,
                  def = "excess",
                  backgType = "modelBased",
                  display = FALSE)
```

```
BMD.Kociba$Results
```

```
##        BMD      BMDL
##   4.795546  1.175081
```

Combining estimates from dose-response models can be done using a meta-analytic approach: We construct a new dataset collecting estimates and standard errors for BMD from all (here only two) studies. Standard errors are calculated from BMDL knowing these were based on Wald-type confidence intervals.

```
step2Data <- data.frame(BMD = c(BMD.NTP$Results[1],
                                BMD.Kociba$Results[1]),
                        SE = c(BMD.NTP$SE,
                               BMD.Kociba$SE))
```

For the meta-analysis approach, we use the package *metafor*. In meta-analysis, estimation involves weights, which depend on the standard errors as well as the between-study variation. If we want to put more weight on the new dataset, we can instead provide our own weights. For our current data example, we choose to assign less weight to older studies.

```
step2Data$my.weights <- c(1,0.5)
```

```
meta.m1 <- rma(BMD,
               SE^2,
               data = step2Data,
               weights = my.weights,
               level = 0.9)

meta.m1

##
## Random-Effects Model (k = 2; tau^2 estimator: REML)
##
## tau^2 (estimated amount of total heterogeneity): 178.1907
##      (SE = 258.1913)
## tau (square root of estimated tau^2 value):       13.3488
## I^2 (total heterogeneity / total variability):   97.60%
## H^2 (total variability / sampling variability):  41.70
##
## Test for Heterogeneity:
## Q(df = 1) = 41.7000, p-val < .0001
##
## Model Results:
##
## estimate       se     zval     pval    ci.lb    ci.ub
##  17.5346  10.0634   1.7424   0.0814   0.9818  34.0874  .
##
## ---
## Signif. codes: 0 '***' 0.001 '**' 0.01 '*' 0.05 '.' 0.1 ' ' 1
```

By combing the two studies we find that the estimated BMD is equal to 17.53 ng/kg and the corresponding estimated BMDL is equal to 0.98 ng/kg.

6.2   Continuous dose-response data

For continuous responses, things are more complicated as there is no longer a natural probability scale for the response between 0 and 1. One possible straightforward definition of BMD is to base it upon a relative calculation (Murrell *et al.*, 1998):

$$BMR = \frac{f(BMD, \beta) - f(0, \beta)}{f(\infty, \beta) - f(0, \beta)} \tag{6.3}$$

This definition resembles that of effective doses for continuous dose-response data. However, the definition does not incorporate any background level due to the occurrence of adverse events.

The so-called hybrid approach leads to more sensible definitions incorporating a background level (Gaylor and Slikker, 1990; Kodell and West, 1993; Budtz-Jørgensen et al., 2001). Basically, the hybrid approach defines the BMD as the dose corresponding to a predefined increase in risk/probability of falling below (or exceeding) a certain cut-off value on the response scale. The cut-off, x_0, dividing values of the continuous response into ranges of normal and adverse values may be defined in several ways. It may be based on expert knowledge or using a certain percentile in the distribution of the unexposed population.

Assuming a normal distribution for the unexposed population, the background risk, p_0, which is the probability of experiencing an adverse event for a member of the unexposed population, can be calculated as follows:

$$p_0 = 1 - \Phi\left(\frac{x_0 - f(0, \beta)}{\sigma}\right) \tag{6.4}$$

for a dose-response model function f, described by parameters β and Φ, which denotes the cumulative distribution function of a standard normal distribution. Similarly, we consider the probability of an adverse response in an exposed population. Based on the hybrid approach, the BMD, defined in terms of additional risk, is given as the solution to the following equation:

$$BMR = 1 - \Phi\left(\frac{x_0 - f(BMD, \beta)}{\sigma}\right) - p_0 \tag{6.5}$$

Likewise, for excess risk, BMD is the solution to the equation:

$$BMR = \frac{1 - \Phi\left(\frac{x_0 - f(BMD, \beta)}{\sigma}\right) - p_0}{1 - p_0} \tag{6.6}$$

With these definitions in place we consider two examples.

6.2.1 Toxicity of copper in an ecosystem with giant kelp

In an ecotoxicological study of heavy metal contamination, Giant kelp, *Mactocystis pyrifera*, was exposed to different concentrations of copper. Eight different concentrations were used with up to 5 replicates per concentration. The response was the length of the germination tubes, the shorter the tube the more toxic was the heavy metal contamination. Data are taken from Chapman et al. (1995).

```
head(GiantKelp)
```

```
##     tubeLength dose
## 1        19.58  0.0
```

```
## 2        18.75   0.0
## 3        19.14   0.0
## 4        16.50   0.0
## 5        17.93   0.0
## 6        18.26   5.6
```

A four-parameter log-logistic model is fitted to data.

```
kelp.m1 <- drm(tubeLength ~ dose,
               data = GiantKelp,
               fct = LL.4())
```

As expected we see a decreasing trend in the length of the germination tubes with an increasing concentration of copper in the water environment (Figure 6.4).

```
plot(kelp.m1,
     type = "all",
     broken = TRUE,
     xlab = expression(paste("Copper ", mu, "g/L",sep="")),
     ylab = "Length germination tube (mm)")
```

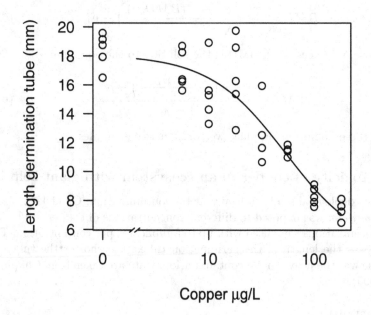

FIGURE 6.4
Four-parameter log-logistic model fitted to the dataset GiantKelp.

To estimate the BMD and corresponding BMDL, we first need to define what an adverse event is. Such a definition could be based on expert knowledge. For instance, a length of germination tube shorter than 14 mm could imply inability to function properly. Then we would use 14 mm as the cut-off. The BMD and corresponding BMDL, associated with a BMR = 0.1, can now be found using the function bmd(). We specify the background risk based on an absolute level of the response, which is length of the germination tubes. This means that we specify the background using the argument backgType = "absolute".

```
bmd(kelp.m1,
    0.1,
    backgType = "absolute",
    backg = 14,
    def = "hybridAdd")
```

```
##       BMD       BMDL
## 12.30724 5.248608
```

We could also have used the cut-off for dichotomizing the continuous response variable. Then everything would seemingly become simpler in the sense that we could stick to the binomial dose-response model where BMD is perhaps more conveniently defined.

```
GiantKelp$tubeLengthBin <- with(GiantKelp,
                                ifelse(tubeLength < 14, 1, 0))
```

```
kelp.m2 <- drm(tubeLengthBin ~ dose,
               data = GiantKelp,
               fct = LL.4(),
               type = "binomial")
```

```
bmd(kelp.m2,
    0.1,
    backgType = "modelBased",
    def = "additional")
```

```
##      BMD       BMDL
## 9.278657 -53.68048
```

The estimated BMD becomes somewhat smaller, but the estimated BMDL becomes much smaller, taking on a negative value. So, by dichotomizing the data, we lose much information. In this example so much information is lost that we in principle are not able to say anything about the BMD; it could be any value.

In practice, a cut-off for defining an adverse event is rarely known. Instead we can use 2 standard deviations (SD) based on the background distribution to define an adverse event. The argument `backType = "hybridSD"` specifies that the background levels should be based on the SD for the control group. The default is to use 2·SD.

```
bmd(kelp.m1,
    0.1,
    backgType = "hybridSD",
    def = "hybridAdd")
```

```
##        BMD       BMDL
## 8.878006 2.542278
```

Finally, looking at the residual plot in Figure 6.5 we may doubt the validity of the assumption of variance homogeneity.

```
plot(resid(kelp.m1) ~ predict(kelp.m1),
    ylab = "Residuals",
    xlab = "Predicted")
abline(h = 0)
```

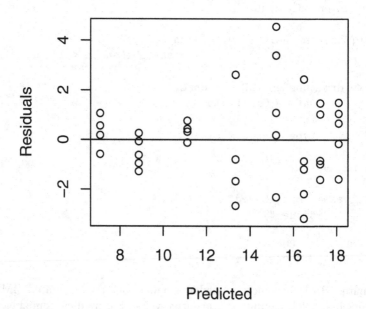

FIGURE 6.5
Residual plot for the four-parameter log-logistic model fitted to the dataset `GiantKelp`.

A simple way to address the apparent model misspecification is to base the BMDL on robust standard errors (see Section A.5 for more details).

```
bmd(kelp.m1,
    0.1,
    backgType = "hybridSD",
    def = "hybridAdd",
    sandwich.vcov = TRUE)

##        BMD      BMDL
## 8.878006 1.275386
```

In this case the robust standard errors are larger and the estimated BMDL becomes smaller.

6.2.2 Toxicity of an antituberculosis drug

Aconiazide is a drug against tuberculosis. Beland *et al.* (1995) reported data from a study examining the systemic toxicity of the drug in male Fisher 344 rats. The response was the weight change over a 6-month period with one of four daily doses received by gavage.

A four-parameter log-logistic model fits the data adequately as seen in Figure 6.6.

```
aconiazide.m1 <- drm(weightChange ~ dose,
                data = aconiazide,
                fct = LL.4())
```

The summary output is shown below.

```
summary(aconiazide.m1)

##
## Model fitted: Log-logistic (ED50 as parameter) (4 parms)
##
## Parameter estimates:
##
##                 Estimate Std. Error t-value p-value
## b:(Intercept)    1.11216    0.45229  2.4589 0.01737 *
## c:(Intercept)  -46.62436  821.98122 -0.0567 0.95499
## d:(Intercept)  360.39895    4.96987 72.5168 < 2e-16 ***
## e:(Intercept) 1106.79578 3076.78714  0.3597 0.72054
## ---
## Signif. codes: 0 '***' 0.001 '**' 0.01 '*' 0.05 '.' 0.1 ' ' 1
##
## Residual standard error:
##
##   18.72333 (51 degrees of freedom)
```

```
plot(aconiazide.m1,
     broken = TRUE,
     type = "all",
     xlab = "Aconiazide (mg/kg)",
     ylab = "Weight change (g)")
```

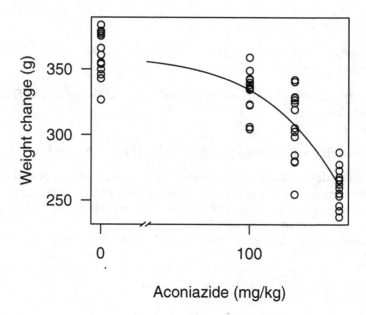

FIGURE 6.6
Four-parameter log-logistic model fitted to the dataset `aconiazide`.

We use again the hybrid approach to estimate the BMD and BMDL for a BMR = 0.05 but this time the background risk is based on a 3 SD cut-off. As an alternative to the Wald-type confidence intervals used in the previous example, we use an inverse regression approach (see Section A.9 and Section A.10). The function `bmd()` is specified as follows.

```
bmd(aconiazide.m1,
    0.05,
    backgType = "hybridSD",
    backg = 3,
    def = "hybridAdd",
    interval = "inv")
```

```
##        BMD       BMDL
## 97.61672 68.73968
```

While the four-parameter log-logistic model provided a good fit to data, it could be argued that a three-parameter model with a lower limit fixed at 0 is biologically justifiable because extremely high doses of aconiazide may cause the rat to die immediately, resulting in a weight change of 0 g. We also note that the estimated parameter c in the above model fit was negative, indicating that there is no information in the data to estimate this parameter. Below we fit this reduced model and evaluate how much the estimated BMD and BMDL are changed.

```
aconiazide.m2 <- drm(weightChange ~ dose,
                     data = aconiazide,
                     fct = LL.3())
```

```
bmd(aconiazide.m2,
    0.05,
    backgType = "hybridSD",
    backg = 3,
    def = "hybridAdd",
    interval = "inv")
```

```
##       BMD      BMDL
## 97.24473 75.20937
```

The hybrid approach based on the three-parameter log-logistic model fit results in an estimated BMD of similar magnitude as before but with a higher estimated BMDL, reflecting that fewer parameters were fitted. This example reinforces that the choice of model function is crucial as it may affect the BMDL.

6.3 Model averaging

Interpolation in a dose region with little or no data is highly dependent on the fit of a dose-response model. In studies estimating BMD and BMDL the choice of dose-response model describing data can be crucial for the conclusions (Budtz-Jørgensen *et al.*, 2001; Sand *et al.*, 2002). To increase robustness of the benchmark dose approach, it has been proposed to evaluate several models and subsequently select the best model determined by means of some goodness-of-fit criterion (Slob, 2002). However, this procedure does not incorporate the uncertainty pertaining to the model selection process and results based on a "best fitting" model found by a model selection procedure may result in biased estimates of BMD and too high (non-protecting) estimates of BMDL (West *et al.*, 2012; Ringblom *et al.*, 2014). As a consequence, it has been repeatedly advocated to use model averaging for estimation of BMD and BMDL (Kang *et al.*, 2000; Bailer *et al.*, 2005; Wheeler and Bailer, 2007; Faes *et al.*, 2007; Namata *et al.*, 2008; Wheeler *et al.*, 2008; Jensen and Ritz, 2015).

Model averaging means forming a model-averaged estimated BMD as a weighted average of the estimates of BMD obtained from all separately fitted candidate models. Estimation of BMD through model averaging implies that flexibility of candidate models to some extent compensates for lack of data. Specifically, for K candidate models and assuming weights w_k such that $\sum_k w_k = 1$, the formula of the weighted average is shown below.

$$\text{BMD}_{\text{MA}} = \sum_{k=1}^{K} w_k \text{BMD}_k$$

One choice of weights is the AIC weights defined as follows:

$$w_k = \frac{\exp(-\text{AIC}_k)}{\sum_{k=1}^{K} \exp(-\text{AIC}_k)}$$

The above definition of a model-averaged estimated BMD is straightforward to estimate. In contrast, it is more complicated to estimate the corresponding BMDL; it has been the subject of much methodological research. Current practice is to use either a type of bootstrap approach (Wheeler and Bailer, 2007; Wheeler *et al.*, 2008; Buckley *et al.*, 2009; Moon *et al.*, 2013), a simple average of estimates of BMDL from the candidate models (Kang *et al.*, 2000), or an approximation based on a variance inequality (Buckland *et al.*, 1997; Faes *et al.*, 2007; Jensen and Ritz, 2015).

An alternative to averaging estimates of BMD is to make a weighted average of all candidate model fits, i.e., an average of the estimated dose-response curves (Wheeler and Bailer, 2007). Below we provide examples of both model averaging approaches.

6.3.1 Pathogens in food revisited

We return to the *Echovirus 12* data from Subsection 6.1.1. Recall that we previously fitted a two-parameter log-logistic model to data. However, other models may also provide a reasonable or perhaps even better fit to the data. Therefore, we fit two additional models to the same data: a two-parameter log-normal model and a two-parameter Weibull model.

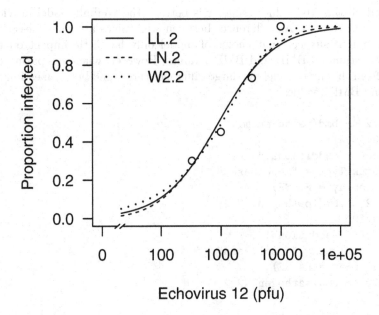

FIGURE 6.7
Three different two-parameter models fitted to the dataset **echovirus**.

```
pathogen.LN.2 <- drm(infected/total ~ dose,
                    weights = total, data = echovirus,
                    fct = LN.2(), type = "binomial")

pathogen.W2.2 <- drm(infected/total ~ dose,
                    weights = total, data = echovirus,
                    fct = W2.2(), type = "binomial")
```

Figure 6.7 indicates that the Weibull model may be the better choice in this case (**R** lines for the plot are provided in Subsection C.2.1).

Besides the visual assessment of the different model fits, AIC may also be used for comparing the model fits.

```
pathogen.AIC <- AIC(pathogen.m1, pathogen.LN.2, pathogen.W2.2)
pathogen.AIC

##              df      AIC
## pathogen.m1   2 18.31155
## pathogen.LN.2 2 17.99485
## pathogen.W2.2 2 16.80155
```

Based on the AIC values (smaller is better), the Weibull model provides the better fit to data. As differences between AIC values are small (less than 10), one might suspect that choice of model only has little impact on the resulting estimated BMD and BMDL values. However, when comparing the results from the three model fits, large differences are found between estimated BMD and BMDL values.

```
bmd.LL.2 <- bmd(pathogen.m1,
      0.10,
      def = "additional",
      backgType = "modelBased",
      display = FALSE)
bmd.LN.2 <- bmd(pathogen.LN.2,
      0.10,
      def = "additional",
      backgType = "modelBased",
      display = FALSE)
bmd.W2.2 <- bmd(pathogen.W2.2,
      0.10,
      def = "additional",
      backgType = "modelBased",
      display = FALSE)
```

```
bmd.LL.2$Results
```

```
##        BMD      BMDL
##    90.32084  10.0272
```

```
bmd.LN.2$Results
```

```
##        BMD      BMDL
##    102.3873  19.13779
```

```
bmd.W2.2$Results
```

```
##      BMD        BMDL
##    60.85477  -5.673325
```

Notice that the BMDL estimated from the Weibull model is –5.67. A negative estimated BMDL is not meaningful since a dose cannot be < 0. In practice, a negative value could be truncated at 0, meaning that we cannot be sure that any dose above 0 result in an added risk less than 10%. The possibility of getting negative values is a drawback of using Wald-type confidence intervals for estimating BMDL. An alternative approach is to use inverse regression. Estimating BMD and BMDL using inverse regression results in positive estimates for all 3 models.

```
bmd.LL.2.inv <- bmd(pathogen.m1, 0.10, def = "additional",
      backgType = "modelBased", interval="inv", display = FALSE)
bmd.LN.2.inv <- bmd(pathogen.LN.2, 0.10, def = "additional",
      backgType = "modelBased", interval="inv", display = FALSE)
bmd.W2.2.inv <- bmd(pathogen.W2.2, 0.10, def = "additional",
      backgType = "modelBased", interval="inv", display = FALSE)


bmd.LL.2.inv$Results

##        BMD       BMDL
##   90.32084  40.08553

bmd.LN.2.inv$Results

##        BMD       BMDL
##   102.3873  49.28374

bmd.W2.2.inv$Results

##        BMD       BMDL
##   60.85477  22.06095
```

The Weibull model still results in a much lower estimated BMDL compared to the other models. In this case, both the choice of dose-response model function and how to derive the BMDL really matters for the conclusion.

Instead of reporting the BMDL from a single "best fitting," model as we did above, we can use model averaging. Choosing AIC weights results in the following weights, which show that all three models will contribute to the weighted average.

```
AICWeights <- exp(-pathogen.AIC$AIC) /
                  sum(exp(-pathogen.AIC$AIC))
AICWeights

## [1] 0.1449426 0.1989451 0.6561123
```

Model averaging can be carried out using the function bmdMA(), which as the first argument, takes a list of the models. The second argument specifies the weights to be used. These can be directly specified by the user or indirectly as shown below. Arguments for how BMD and BMR are specified follow the style of the function bmd(). Finally, we need to specify how to estimate the BMDL. The choice type = "Kang" results in an estimated BMDL being the simple weighted average of the estimated BMDL values from the separately fitted candidate models.

```
bmdMA(modelList = list(pathogen.m1,pathogen.LN.2,pathogen.W2.2),
      modelWeights = "AIC",
      bmr = 0.1,
      def = "additional",
      backgType = "modelBased",
      interval = "inv",
      type = "Kang")
```

```
##    BMD_MA   BMDL_MA
## 73.38836 30.08932
```

6.3.2 Toxicity of an antituberculosis drug revisited

We revisit the example on aconiazide from Subsection 6.2.2. In this experiment, only relatively low doses are provided, leaving room for a lot of variation in the high-dose area. Consequently, several models may describe the data adequately. We consider a total of four different three-parameter models; the log-logistic model already fitted to data and the fit saved in the object aconiazide.m1, a log-normal model, and two different Weibull models.

```
aconiazide.LN.3 <- drm(weightChange ~ dose,
                       data = aconiazide, fct = LN.3())
aconiazide.W1.3 <- drm(weightChange ~ dose,
                       data = aconiazide, fct = W1.3())
aconiazide.W2.3 <- drm(weightChange ~ dose,
                       data = aconiazide, fct = W2.3())
```

The four models provide similar fits to data in the low-dose region (Figure 6.8, **R** lines provided in Subsection C.2.2), while deviating more when extrapolating to high doses as seen in Figure 6.9. A model-averaged estimated BMD with the corresponding BMDL being estimated using non-parametric bootstrap may be obtained using bmdMA() with the argument type = "bootstrap". Non-parametric bootstrap means that new datasets are generated by resampling with replacement from the original dataset. As before, we estimate the BMD associated with a BMR = 0.05 using the hybrid approach with a 3 SD cut-off.

```
bmdMA(modelList = list(aconiazide.m2, aconiazide.LN.3,
                       aconiazide.W1.3, aconiazide.W2.3),
      modelWeights = "AIC",
      bmr = 0.05,
      backgType = "hybridSD",
      backg = 3,
      def = "hybridAdd",
      type = "bootstrap")
```

```
##    BMD_MA   BMDL_MA
## 98.46404 70.32581
```

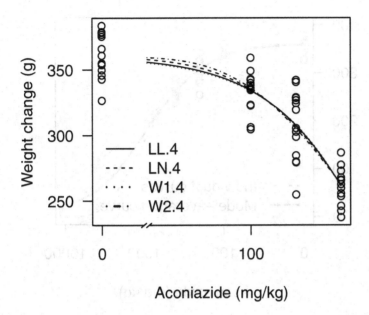

FIGURE 6.8
Four different three-parameter models fitted to the dataset `aconiazide`.

The resulting estimated BMDL is based on the percentile approach, which is more appropriate for the present example with continuous dose-response data than for binomial dose-response data as discussed previously in Subsection 6.3.1. However, we can repeat the analysis using a bias correction approach in order to compare results.

```
bmdMA(modelList = list(aconiazide.m2, aconiazide.LN.3,
                       aconiazide.W1.3, aconiazide.W2.3),
    modelWeights = "AIC",
    bmr=0.05,
    backgType = "hybridSD",
    back = 3,
    def = "hybridAdd",
    type = "bootstrap",
    bootInterval = "BCa")
```

```
##      BMD_MA   BMDL_MA
##    98.46404  70.32321
```

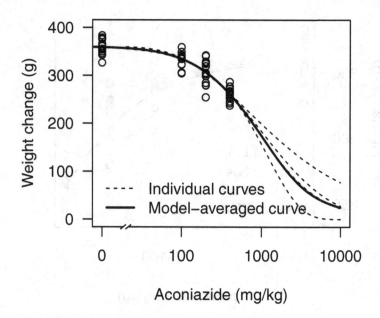

FIGURE 6.9
Four different three-parameter models fitted to the dataset `aconiazide` plotted together with the model-averaged estimated dose-response curve.

The resulting estimated BMDL, 70.32, is close to the estimated BMDL using the percentile approach, 70.33, indicating that the correction made through the BCa procedure was small. In theory, the best option is to always use some kind of adjustment, like BCa, when estimating BMDL using bootstrap. In practice, however, most adjustments add computation time to what may already be a time-consuming analysis. This is especially the case for large datasets.

Finally, we consider model averaging using the approach of averaging the entire fitted dose-response curves. Figure 6.9 shows the model-averaged estimated dose-response curve together with the four individual estimated dose-response curves (**R** lines for the plot are provided in Subsection C.2.2).

Estimating BMD and BMDL based on model averaging of all curves can be achieved using the argument `type = "curve"`.

```
bmdMA(modelList = list(aconiazide.m2, aconiazide.LN.3,
                       aconiazide.W1.3, aconiazide.W2.3),
      modelWeights = "AIC",
```

```
    bmr = 0.05,
    backgType = "hybridSD",
    back = 3,
    def = "hybridAdd",
    type = "curve")

##     BMD_MA  BMDL_MA
##  98.76187 70.72517
```

It is noteworthy that the change of method not only results in a different estimated BMDL but also in a different estimated BMD.

7

Hierarchical nonlinear models

Most dose-response experiments are not designed with a simple random sampling structure for each observation. Hierarchical or multilevel designs are common, collecting observations repeatedly from the same individual or grouping individuals into blocks or subunits, e.g., different assays, animal cages, or laboratories. Any factor that restricts a random sampling design needs to be included in the dose-response model; therefore, for a hierarchical design, the correlation between observations from the same experimental unit needs to be taken into account.

Certain correlation structures may readily be implemented within the framework of *drc*, e.g., correlation that is a function of the dose-response model function (Strodl Andersen *et al.*, 1998). The package *medrc* extends many of the capabilities of *drc* to correlated dose-response data fitted through nonlinear mixed-effects regression models. Specifically, *medrc* utilizes the capabilities of the package *nlme* (Pinheiro and Bates, 2000); additionally, *medrc* offers the same user-friendly interface for estimating and comparing derived ED50 or benchmark dose parameters.

7.1 Normally distributed dose-response data

A simple hierarchical design consists of observing several response values within several groups (x_{ij}, y_{ij}), with $i = 1, \ldots, n_j$ observations within the group $j = 1, \ldots, M$, or in vector notation (x_j, y_j). Then within each group j a separate nonlinear model can be assumed:

$$y_j = f_j\left(x_j, \beta_j\right) + \epsilon_j$$

The effects between the groups are modeled on the level of the individual parameters for each group

$$\beta_j = A_j \tilde{\beta} + B_j b_j$$

where the matrix A_j defines the vector of unknown population parameters $\tilde{\beta}$ and the indicator matrix B_j determines the contribution of each observations to the group effects b_j. Similar to the assumption of normally distributed

145

residuals $\epsilon_{ij} \sim N\left(0, \sigma^2\right)$, we can assume that the group effects also follow a normal distribution

$$b_j \sim N\left(\mathbf{0}, \mathbf{\Psi}\right)$$

summarizing their effect on each parameter as a variance component. With this assumption of modeling the individual parameters as random effects, the variance on the scale of each parameter is decomposed into between- and within-group variability. Further, the parametrization of the individual effects through variance components allows us to estimate population effects from individual samples with different content of information, e.g., unbalanced designs with different numbers of observations for each individual or different dose allocation.

Estimating the unknown parameters in the hierarchical nonlinear model by maximum likelihood is a challenge. In Appendix A.7 two-stage estimators for β are discussed.

7.2   The R package medrc

A full maximum likelihood and restricted maximum likelihood implementation of nonlinear mixed-effects models is available in the **R** package *nlme* (Pinheiro and Bates, 2000). Parameters are estimated using the Lindstrom-Bates algorithm with the function `nlme()`, where the user has to specify the nonlinear function and the design matrices for fixed and random effects using a formula interface.

For simple hierarchical dose-response experiments, the package *medrc* provides a user-friendly interface similar to the function `drm()`, using the package *nlme* in the background. All the functionality of the package *drc* to estimate and compare effective dose levels is extended to hierarchical models, but restricted to the use of only a single fixed-effects grouping factor.

```
library(devtools)
install_github("DoseResponse/drcData")
install_github("DoseResponse/drc")
install_github("DoseResponse/medrc")
```

```
library(medrc)
```

A more flexible two-stage estimation approach is available with the function `metadrm()`, which combines estimates from individual `drm()` fits using the **R** package *metafor* (Viechtbauer, 2010). As a restriction, the function `metadrm()` can include only a single random grouping factor in the second stage.

7.2.1 In vitro effects of the fungicide vinclozolin

Nellemann *et al.* (2003) carried out experiments to assess the in vitro effects of the fungicide vinclozolin. Chinese hamster ovary cells were exposed to nine different concentrations of vinclozolin (in μM) for 22 hours and the resulting luminescence effects were recorded in an AR reporter gene assay (in luminescence units). The basic dose-response experiment was repeated 6 times on different days. The same nine concentrations were used in all six assays. However, one observation was missing in one assay.

```
head(vinclozolin)
```

```
##    exper  conc effect
## 1 10509 0.000   1003
## 2 10509 0.025    908
## 3 10509 0.050    997
## 4 10509 0.100    744
## 5 10509 0.200    567
## 6 10509 0.390    314
```

A plausible biological assumption was that no signal would be observed for very high fungicide concentrations, indicating that a three-parameter log-logistic model (Section B.1.1.1) with a lower asymptote at 0 would be a realistic model for the data. The individual effects of each repeated experiment can be added as normally distributed random effects onto all three parameters: the slope, asymptote, and ED50.

The model coefficients can be estimated with the two-stage approach, using the function `metadrm()`. The interface uses the same arguments as the `drm()` function in package *drc*, but additionally, the second stage grouping needs to be defined by a factor that is included with the argument `ind`. The random effect variance-covariance is defined with the argument `struct`, using the default of an unstructured matrix, estimating all random effect variances and covariances.

```
metamod <- metadrm(effect ~ conc,
                   data = vinclozolin,
                   fct = LL.3(),
                   ind = exper,
                   struct = "UN")
summary(metamod)
```

```
##
## Two-stage meta-analysis dose-response model
## Model fitted: Log-logistic (ED50 as parameter) with lower
##      limit at 0
##
## Call:
```

```
## metadrm(formula = effect ~ conc, fct = LL.3(), ind = exper,
##      data = vinclozolin, struct = "UN")
##
## Variance estimates:
##                    estim        sqrt
## tau^2.1           0.0316      0.1779
## tau^2.2      687777.9233    829.3238
## tau^2.3           0.0069      0.0830
##
##                  rho.b:(I   rho.d:(I   rho.e:(I
## b:(Intercept)           1    -0.8745     0.9315
## d:(Intercept)     -0.8745          1    -0.6382
## e:(Intercept)      0.9315    -0.6382          1
##
##
## Coefficients:
##                   Estimate     Std.Err   t value   Pr(>|t|)
## b:(Intercept) 5.4042e-01  7.8816e-02    6.8568  5.444e-06 ***
## d:(Intercept) 1.9684e+03  3.4107e+02    5.7711  3.692e-05 ***
## e:(Intercept) 1.0312e-01  3.6090e-02    2.8573    0.01199 *
## ---
## Signif. codes: 0 '***' 0.001 '**' 0.01 '*' 0.05 '.' 0.1 ' ' 1
```

The estimates for the population parameters, slope (b), asymptote (d), and
ED50 (e), are presented in the Coefficients section of the summary output together with corresponding standard errors and hypothesis tests for each
coefficient being different to zero. The Variance estimates section contains
the estimated between-assay variance on the scale of each of the three parameters, together with the estimated standard deviation as the square root of
the variance.

Functions to obtain the effective dose in the package *drc* can be directly
applied to the *medrc* object; here, we are looking at the estimated ED25,
ED50, and ED75 and their corresponding confidence intervals derived by the
delta method.

```
ED(metamod, respLev = c(25, 50, 75), interval = "delta")

##
## Estimated effective doses
##
##           Estimate  Std. Error       Lower       Upper
## e::25    0.0135045   0.0083568  -0.0043075   0.0313165
## e::50    0.1031208   0.0360900   0.0261969   0.1800448
## e::75    0.7874328   0.1531680   0.4609629   1.1139026
```

The effective dose estimates are derived from the estimated population parameters and, therefore, these estimates may also be interpreted as population averages.

As an alternative to the two-stage approach, the full likelihood can be maximized with the Lindstrom-Bates algorithm using function `medrm()`.

```
mod <- medrm(effect ~ conc,
             data = vinclozolin,
             fct = LL.3(),
             random = b + d + e ~ 1|exper,
             start = c(0.5, 2000, 0.1))
summary(mod)

## Nonlinear mixed-effects model fit by maximum likelihood
##   Model: effect ~ meLL.3(conc, b, d, e)
## Data: data
##        AIC      BIC    logLik
##    701.486 721.1889 -340.743
##
## Random effects:
##  Formula: list(b ~ 1, d ~ 1, e ~ 1)
##  Level: exper
##  Structure: General positive-definite, Log-Cholesky
##      parametrization
##          StdDev      Corr
## b        0.15226038  b        d
## d      758.87840398 -0.893
## e        0.06970198  0.859 -0.537
## Residual 100.09082654
##
## Fixed effects: b + d + e ~ 1
##        Value Std.Error DF  t-value p-value
## b     0.5382    0.0706 45 7.624322  0.0000
## d 1987.3111  321.4787 45 6.181782  0.0000
## e     0.1014    0.0322 45 3.144618  0.0029
##  Correlation:
##    b      d
## d -0.819
## e  0.812 -0.517
##
## Standardized Within-Group Residuals:
##         Min          Q1         Med          Q3         Max
## -1.94006282 -0.51813906 -0.09170977  0.49904958  2.20590189
##
## Number of Observations: 53
## Number of Groups: 6
```

The output is structured in the same way as for the `metadrc` object with the population parameter estimates in the `Fixed effects` section and the between-assay standard deviation estimates in the `Random effects` section. The pairwise correlation between random effects are presented as the lower triangular part of the correlation matrix directly beside the estimated variance components.

The function `ED()` can be directly applied to the mixed-effects model object:

```
ED(mod, respLev = c(25, 50, 75), interval = "delta")

##
## Estimated effective doses
##
##             Estimate Std. Error      Lower      Upper
## e:1:25     0.0131600  0.0071288 -0.0011895  0.0275096
## e:1:50     0.1013562  0.0313061  0.0383402  0.1643722
## e:1:75     0.7806264  0.1410174  0.4967731  1.0644798
```

We obtain almost similar effective dose-estimates as for the two-stage estimation approach; only the standard error estimates are a bit smaller for the full maximum likelihood method.

7.2.2   Inhibition of photosynthesis in spinach

Streibig *et al.* (1999) investigated the inhibition of photosynthesis in response to two synthetic photosystem II inhibitors, the herbicides diuron and bentazon. In an experiment, the effect of oxygen consumption of thylakoid membranes (chloroplasts) from spinach was measured after incubation with the synthetic inhibitors. Five assays, three treated with bentazon and two with diuron, were used. For each assay, six increasing herbicide concentrations were applied together with a negative control, using different dose ranges on a logarithmic scale for the two treatments to encompass the whole dose-response range based on preliminary experiments.

```
spinach$CURVE <- as.factor(spinach$CURVE)
head(spinach)

##   CURVE HERBICIDE DOSE    SLOPE
## 1     1  bentazon 0.00 1.81295
## 2     1  bentazon 0.00 1.86704
## 3     1  bentazon 0.00 1.95606
## 4     1  bentazon 0.62 1.39073
## 5     1  bentazon 0.62 1.15721
## 6     1  bentazon 0.62 1.06126
```

For the comparison of the two herbicides, dose-response curves were fitted assuming a three-parameter log-logistic model (Section B.1.1.1) with a separate set of slope, upper asymptote, and ED50 parameters for each of the two treatments. Individual assay effects were included on the slope, upper asymptote, and ED50 parameters to model the between-assay variability in the different model scales. Using the information about the between-assay variability is especially advantageous as the dose levels for the two herbicides did not cover the same dose range.

The `curveid` argument in function `drm()` defines a set of model parameters for every level of a categorical predictor variable, which groups together observations within an individual. When we want to estimate a separate set of parameters for each herbicide, we need to extend the indicator matrix A_j adding indicator variables for multiple curves on the between-individual level of the second stage. The `metadrm()` function contains an argument `cid2` that lets us define a curve identifier to group specific individual curves together. Similar to the argument `pmodels` in function `drm()`, the argument `pms2` allows us to define different fixed-effects design matrices for each population parameter on the between-individual level of the second stage.

```
metaspinach <- metadrm(SLOPE ~ DOSE,
                       data = spinach,
                       fct = LL.3(),
                       ind = CURVE,
                       cid2 = HERBICIDE,
                       struct = "UN")
summary(metaspinach)

##
## Two-stage meta-analysis dose-response model
## Model fitted: Log-logistic (ED50 as parameter) with lower
##      limit at 0
##
## Call:
## metadrm(formula = SLOPE ~ DOSE, fct = LL.3(), ind = CURVE,
##      data = spinach, cid2 = HERBICIDE, struct = "UN")
##
## Variance estimates:
##              estim    sqrt
## tau^2.1     0.0005  0.0221
## tau^2.2     0.1856  0.4308
## tau^2.3     0.0000  0.0009
##
##                  rho.b:(I  rho.d:(I  rho.e:(I
## b:(Intercept)           1   1.0000   -1.0000
## d:(Intercept)      1.0000        1   -1.0000
## e:(Intercept)     -1.0000  -1.0000         1
```

```
##
##
## Coefficients:
##              Estimate   Std.Err  t value   Pr(>|t|)
## b:bentazon  0.5021927  0.0252658  19.8764  9.590e-09 ***
## b:diuron    1.6572431  0.1154678  14.3524  1.654e-07 ***
## d:bentazon  1.3091412  0.2495357   5.2463  0.0005303 ***
## d:diuron    1.9858581  0.3056731   6.4967  0.0001119 ***
## e:bentazon  1.7452319  0.1716524  10.1672  3.116e-06 ***
## e:diuron    0.2086242  0.0091462  22.8100  2.840e-09 ***
## ---
## Signif. codes:  0 '***' 0.001 '**' 0.01 '*' 0.05 '.' 0.1 ' ' 1
```

The correlation estimates at the boundary of the parameter space of -1 and 1 indicate that there might not be enough information available to estimate the full unstructured random effect covariance matrix Ψ. The `struct` argument allows choosing a different correlation structure, e.g., a scaled compound-symmetry or diagonal structure instead.

The curves for the two different herbicides can be compared by the ratio of effective dose levels. The `EDcomp()` function is used to compare the population estimates of the ED15, ED50, and ED85.

```
EDcomp(metaspinach,
       percVec = c(15, 50, 85),
       percMat = rbind(c(1, 1),
                       c(2, 2),
                       c(3, 3)),
       interval = "delta")
```

```
##
## Estimated ratios of effect doses
##
##                         Estimate    Lower      Upper
## bentazon/diuron:15/15    0.75332   0.38388    1.12275
## bentazon/diuron:50/50    8.36543   6.32764   10.40322
## bentazon/diuron:85/85   92.89634  47.22788  138.56480
```

The herbicide Diuron shows an effective inhibition at much lower dose levels compared to Bentazon; although, a comparison of relative effective dose levels is difficult to interpret with large differences between the upper asymptotes.

The same three-parameter log-logistic model can be fitted with the `medrm()` function, using a full likelihood approach.

```
modspinach <- medrm(SLOPE ~ DOSE,
                    curveid = b + d + e ~ HERBICIDE,
```

```
                data = spinach,
                fct = LL.3(),
                random = b + d + e ~ 1|CURVE,
                start = c(0.5, 1, 1.5, 1.5, 1.5, 0.3))
round(summary(modspinach$fit)$tTable[, 1:2], 3)

##                         Value Std.Error
## b.HERBICIDEbentazon  0.503     0.028
## b.HERBICIDEdiuron    1.659     0.087
## d.HERBICIDEbentazon  1.311     0.197
## d.HERBICIDEdiuron    1.986     0.241
## e.HERBICIDEbentazon  1.848     0.205
## e.HERBICIDEdiuron    0.209     0.007
```

The effective doses can be compared in a similar way as for the two-stage estimation, resulting in comparable estimates.

```
EDcomp(modspinach,
       percVec = c(15, 50, 85),
       percMat = rbind(c(1, 1),
                       c(2, 2),
                       c(3, 3)),
       interval = "fieller")

##
## Estimated ratios of effect doses
##
##                          Estimate    Lower     Upper
## bentazon/diuron:15/15     0.80056   0.39510   1.23745
## bentazon/diuron:50/50     8.86013   6.90605  10.89971
## bentazon/diuron:85/85    98.05904  63.37850 135.24171
```

The construction of the plot in Figure 7.1, showing the predicted curves for each individual assay together with the population prediction is shown in Section C.3.1.

7.2.3 Herbicides with auxin effects

Four different herbicides were applied in six different concentrations, either as technical grades material or as commercial formulations to experimental units consisting of five one-week old seedlings (Streibig, 1987). The data consist of the 150 observations of dry weights, each observation being the weight of five plants grown in the same pot. The experiment is replicated three times, each replication with an additional external control of concentration zero.

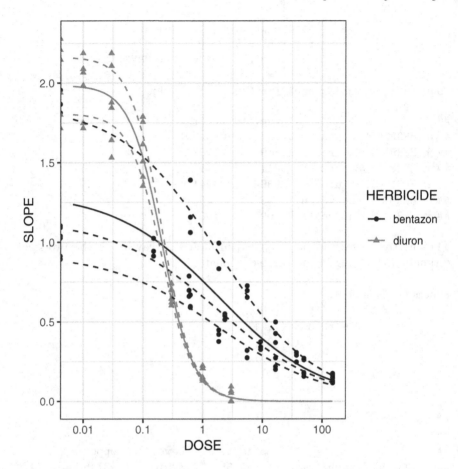

FIGURE 7.1
Scatterplot with the individual assay and population predictions for the two
herbicides bentazon and diuron.

All the eight herbicide preparations have essentially the same mode of
action in the plant; they all act like the plant auxins, which are plant regulators
that affect cell elongation and other essential metabolic pathways.

```
head(auxins)
```

```
##   dryweight  dose replicate herbicide formulation
## 1      1.51 0.000         1   control     control
## 2      1.43 0.000         1   control     control
## 3      0.05 1.000         1      MCPA        tech
## 4      0.06 0.500         1      MCPA        tech
## 5      0.15 0.250         1      MCPA        tech
## 6      0.40 0.125         1      MCPA        tech
```

We assume a three-parameter log-logistic model (Section B.1.1.1) for each individual herbicide within a replicate. Additionally, we assume that the dry weight will approach 0 at high concentrations of the herbicide. The variability between replications is modeled by random replication effects on the upper asymptote parameter. The effects of each herbicide, formulation, and their interaction are modeled as fixed-, main-, and interaction effects of the slope, upper asymptote, and ED50. The external control is joined with the intercept of the first herbicide, estimating all herbicide and interaction effects to this reference group.

As a more complex model is needed to analyze this multifactorial design, we can directly use the function `nlme()` to fit a nonlinear mixed-effects model, where the fixed effects are specified by a user-defined design matrix, copying each predictor variable as a new column into the dataset. The function `model.matrix()` automatically creates dummy-coded predictor variables for the full-factorial combination of herbicide and combination levels. The user-defined design matrix is constructed by extracting certain predictors and adding them as new variables to the dataframe.

The order of the treatment levels is changed to define a reference group; as for the external control, only the information about the upper asymptote parameter is available.

```
auxins$formulation <- relevel(auxins$formulation, ref = "tech")
auxins$herbicide <- relevel(auxins$herbicide, ref = "MCPA")
X <- model.matrix(~ herbicide + formulation +
                    formulation:herbicide, data = auxins)

auxins$h24D <- X[, 3]
auxins$mp <- X[, 4]
auxins$dp <- X[, 5]
auxins$comm <- X[, 7]
auxins$h24Dcomm <- X[, 13]
auxins$mpcomm <- X[, 14]
auxins$dpcomm <- X[, 15]
```

The fixed effect design matrix A_j is defined by including a list for the argument `fixed`, containing a formula for each of the model parameters. The 1 codes for the combined intercept of the common control together with the reference group: the herbicide MCPA as a technical grades material. All further terms denote the effect of each other treatment level to this intercept on the scale of each model parameter.

The function `meLL.3()` is the *medrc* version of the three-parameter log-logistic model, which is compatible for use in the *nlme* package environment.

```
auxmod <- nlme(dryweight ~ meLL.3(dose, b, d, e), data = auxins,
               fixed=list(b ~ 1 + h24D + mp + dp + comm +
                            h24Dcomm + mpcomm + dpcomm,
                          d ~ 1 + h24D + mp + dp + comm +
                            h24Dcomm + mpcomm + dpcomm,
                          e ~ 1 + h24D + mp + dp + comm +
                            h24Dcomm + mpcomm + dpcomm),
               random=d ~ 1|replicate,
               start=c(1.2, rep(0,7), 1, rep(0, 7),
                       0.1, rep(0, 7)))
round(coef(summary(auxmod)), 3)
```

##		Value	Std.Error	DF	t-value	p-value
##	b.(Intercept)	1.827	0.287	124	6.370	0.000
##	b.h24D	0.443	0.609	124	0.727	0.469
##	b.mp	-0.244	0.457	124	-0.533	0.595
##	b.dp	-0.085	0.451	124	-0.188	0.851
##	b.comm	-0.124	0.520	124	-0.239	0.811
##	b.h24Dcomm	0.389	0.957	124	0.406	0.685
##	b.mpcomm	0.315	0.729	124	0.431	0.667
##	b.dpcomm	0.061	0.734	124	0.084	0.933
##	d.(Intercept)	1.278	0.091	124	14.076	0.000
##	d.h24D	-0.145	0.106	124	-1.364	0.175
##	d.mp	-0.047	0.148	124	-0.317	0.751
##	d.dp	-0.069	0.096	124	-0.719	0.473
##	d.comm	0.117	0.267	124	0.440	0.661
##	d.h24Dcomm	-0.081	0.296	124	-0.273	0.785
##	d.mpcomm	0.080	0.339	124	0.237	0.813
##	d.dpcomm	-0.193	0.286	124	-0.674	0.501
##	e.(Intercept)	0.065	0.007	124	9.966	0.000
##	e.h24D	0.069	0.019	124	3.579	0.000
##	e.mp	0.071	0.030	124	2.351	0.020
##	e.dp	0.171	0.035	124	4.934	0.000
##	e.comm	0.009	0.023	124	0.415	0.679
##	e.h24Dcomm	-0.014	0.033	124	-0.443	0.659
##	e.mpcomm	-0.037	0.042	124	-0.880	0.380
##	e.dpcomm	0.303	0.082	124	3.683	0.000

The `Intercept` denotes the estimated slope, asymptote, and ED50 for the MCPA reference as technical grades material. The `h24D`, `mp`, and `dp` coefficients show the largest effects on the ED50 scale; all herbicides as technical grades material reach the ED50 at a higher dose level compared to MCPA. But most obvious is an interaction effect on the ED50 scale (`e.dpcomm`), showing that the commercial formulation of dichlorprop results in an average increase in ED50 compared to the `dp` effect as technical grades material.

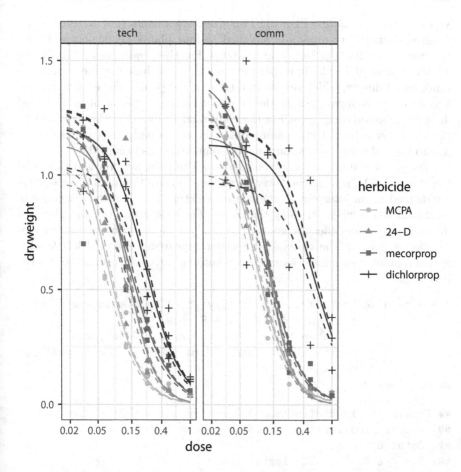

FIGURE 7.2
Scatterplot with the individual replicate and population predictions for four
different herbicides.

The *ggplot2* package is used to draw the scatterplot in Figure 7.2, adding
lines for the predictions on the individual replicate and population level. The
R code to construct the plot can be found in Section C.3.2.

7.2.4 Drought stress resistance in *Brassica oleracea*

The effect of drought stress on *Brassica oleracea* was investigated by selecting
drought-stess-resistant lines out of a population of different double-haploid
(DH) genotypes (Uptmoor *et al.*, 2009). The study was carried out on 48 DH
lines developed from F1 plants of a cross between the rapid cycling Chinese
kale (*Brassica oleracea* var. *alboglabra* (L.H. Bailey) Musil) and broccoli (*Bras-*

sica oleracea var. *italica* Plenck). Two stress treatments (not watered and a watered control) are randomly assigned to four plants per genotype (2 per treatment) resulting in 192 plants in total. For the genotypes 5, 17, 31, and 48, an additional 12 plants (6 per treatment) are included in the completely randomized design, which results in a total of 240 plants. For each plant, the length of the youngest leaf at the beginning of the experiment is measured daily for a period of 16 days. For the additional 12 plants of the 4 genotypes, the leaf water potential was measured as a secondary endpoint (omitted here); due to these destructive measurements, some dropouts occurred.

The growth curves are assumed to follow a three-parameter logistic model (Section B.1.1.1), setting the lower asymptote to zero. Population parameters are defined as an intercept at the control treatment and as the difference in treatment levels when stressing the plants. For each genotype, an individual intercept and stress effect is assumed as random effects with an unstructured covariance matrix. The correlation between repeatedly observed leaf lengths within a plant is estimated assuming an autoregressive AR1 structure for the residuals.

```
brmod <- nlme(LeafLength ~ meL.3(Day, b, d, e), data = broccoli,
              fixed=b + d + e ~ 1 + Stress,
              random=b + d + e ~ 1 + Stress | Genotype,
              correlation = corAR1(form = ~ Day | Genotype/ID),
              start = c(-0.4, 0, 15, 0, 5, 0))
summary(brmod)

## Nonlinear mixed-effects model fit by maximum likelihood
##   Model: LeafLength ~ meL.3(Day, b, d, e)
##   Data: broccoli
##          AIC      BIC   logLik
##     4444.401 4624.581 -2193.2
##
## Random effects:
##  Formula: list(b ~ 1 + Stress, d ~ 1 + Stress, e ~ 1 + Stress)
##  Level: Genotype
##  Structure: General positive-definite, Log-Cholesky
##       parametrization
##                    StdDev      Corr
## b.(Intercept)    0.01370399 b.(In) b.Strs d.(In) d.Strs e.(In)
## b.Stressdrought  0.03609302  0.322
## d.(Intercept)    1.86995266 -0.469  0.123
## d.Stressdrought  1.04427398  0.595 -0.252 -0.839
## e.(Intercept)    0.47151685  0.307  0.306  0.562 -0.517
## e.Stressdrought  0.46963336  0.463  0.196 -0.144  0.574 -0.240
## Residual         1.24750262
##
## Correlation Structure: ARMA(1,0)
```

```
## Formula: ~Day | Genotype/ID
## Parameter estimate(s):
##      Phi1
## 0.9484194
## Fixed effects: b + d + e ~ 1 + Stress
##                     Value  Std.Error   DF    t-value p-value
## b.(Intercept)    -0.366859 0.00626349 3636 -58.57106       0
## b.Stressdrought  -0.067694 0.01163874 3636  -5.81630       0
## d.(Intercept)   14.044417  0.29914816 3636  46.94803       0
## d.Stressdrought -3.267275  0.22960524 3636 -14.22997       0
## e.(Intercept)    5.268797  0.09833708 3636  53.57894       0
## e.Stressdrought -1.442174  0.12301961 3636 -11.72312       0
##  Correlation:
##                   b.(In) b.Strs d.(In) d.Strs e.(In)
## b.Stressdrought  -0.433
## d.(Intercept)     0.076 -0.060
## d.Stressdrought  -0.149  0.254 -0.734
## e.(Intercept)     0.060  0.103  0.369 -0.261
## e.Stressdrought   0.098  0.020 -0.085  0.222 -0.495
##
## Standardized Within-Group Residuals:
##        Min          Q1        Med         Q3        Max
## -5.59627518 -0.58080992 -0.03044674 0.58513286 4.72865998
##
## Number of Observations: 3689
## Number of Groups: 48
```

The summary output shows the estimated population parameters as fixed effects for the control group (intercept), and the difference between parameters for drought stress plants compared to the control. The estimated negative population effects indicate a slower growth with a smaller slope and the inflection point being located at an earlier time. Additionally, the estimated effect for the asymptote shows that the drought stress treatment results in smaller plants. On the scale of each of these parameters, the between-genotype variability is estimated; the genotype standard deviation is presented in the Random effects section together with the pairwise correlation coefficients. The dependency between residuals from a single plant is parametrized as the coefficient of the autoregressive AR1 structure. The estimate of the coefficient is near one, indicating highly correlated residuals within a plant.

Additionally, the predicted random effects can be obtained with the function ranef() or alternatively the linear function of fixed and random effects with the function coef() (not shown here). Instead, we can visualize the genotype-stress interaction by plotting the predicted leaf lengths on the level of each genotype-stress combination in Figure 7.3. The corresponding **R** code can be found in Section C.3.3.

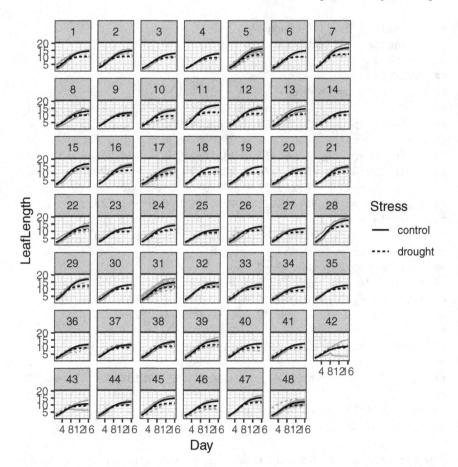

FIGURE 7.3
Plant-specific growth curve predictions, comparing drought-stressed broccoli plants vs. a watered control for each genotype.

The drought stress mainly has an effect on the upper asymptote parameter, that is, the stressed plants are smaller than the watered plants. But we can also see a large negative correlation between the genotype-specific stress effects and the genotype-specific asymptote at the control; hence, genotypes with larger leaves also show the larger response to the drought stress treatment.

Appendix A

Estimation

Once a suitable dose-response model function has been found, the next step is to choose a suitable estimation procedure, which should ideally exploit the type of response as much as possible.

Least squares estimation, which is a special case of maximum likelihood estimation, should be used for continuous response variables that are approximately normally distributed with the same standard deviation for all doses (variance homogeneity) (Meister and den Brink, 2000). Section A.1 below provides more details. More general maximum likelihood estimation involving distributional assumptions different from the normal distribution, may be more appropriate in case the response is binary, a sum of binary variables (Piegorsch and Bailer, 2005, pp. 172-179), or a count with a substantial portion of zeros (Kerr and Meador, 1996; Ritz and Van der Vliet, 2009). More details are provided in Section A.2 below. In practice, least squares estimation is often applied also for responses that are not normally distributed. This approach makes sub-optimal use of the information available in the data, often resulting in a loss in efficiency seen as unnecessary large standard errors (Szöcs and Schäfer, 2015). Therefore, it is important to ensure alignment between the type of response and the estimation procedure used.

To deal with model misspecification the results from maximum likelihood estimation or even the entire estimation procedure may be modified (see Section A.3 on transformations, Section A.4 on robust estimation, and Section A.5 on sandwich variance estimators).

Constrained estimation may be needed in case certain restrictions have to be enforced for certain parameters (see Section A.6). However, surprisingly, in most cases unconstrained estimation will suffice, i.e., no bounds need to be imposed on ranges of any parameters even though ranges for some parameters may be restricted (e.g., ED50/LD50 has to be non-negative), as usually reasonable parameter estimates will be obtained if data carry sufficient information about the parameters. Unreasonable parameter estimates often imply lack of information. It can also happen that the estimation procedure is not successful in finding the optimal parameter estimates. For dose-response analysis such problems often happen due to poor choice of starting values for the parameter estimates: the estimation procedure needs to be provided with good starting values when searching for the optimal parameter estimates. The package *drc* relies heavily on self-starter routines that compute data-driven starting values. Section A.8 explains the idea in more detail.

Estimation of the model parameters or any derived parameters utilizes the entire dose-response data. For some specific parameters, observations may still contribute in an unequal way, e.g., for a decreasing dose-response relationship the estimated upper limit at dose 0 will be mostly influenced by the low-dose range response values, although all response values will contribute to the corresponding standard error (at least in case variance homogeneity is assumed). The uncertainty on parameter estimates is described by means of standard errors or confidence intervals (see Section A.9).

For dose-response analysis, it is of particular interest to estimate effective doses through inverse regression: assuming a given response value and then deriving the corresponding mean dose value. This is the opposite operation of prediction where a mean response is predicted for a given dose. There are various ways to estimate effective doses and the corresponding standard errors. Section A.10 provides details on the different approaches implemented in *drc*.

A.1 Nonlinear least squares

Assume that $x_1, \ldots, x_n$ are the dose values and $y_1, \ldots, y_n$ the corresponding observed responses (assuming a sample size of n). The nonlinear least squares estimates are obtained by minimizing the following sum of squares:

$$\sum_{i=1}^{n} w_i^2 \{y_i - f(x_i, \beta)\}^2 \tag{A.1}$$

where w_i's are user-specified weights (often left unspecified, i.e., equal to 1). β is the vector of all model parameters, i.e., the parameters b, c, d, ... of Appendix B.

In `drm()`, weights are specified through the argument `weights` and they should be on the same scale as the response, e.g., expressed as standard deviations and not empirical variances. Weights may be used for addressing variance heterogeneity in the response. However, the transform-both-sides approach should be preferred instead of using often very imprecisely determined weights.

Equation (A.1) has to be solved numerically in an iterative manner. One approach is to use iteratively weighted least squares as is done in `nls()`, which is part of the standard installation of **R** (Ritz and Streibig, 2008). Another approach is to use a general-purpose minimizer directly, as in `drm()` where `optim()` is used in combination with some pre-scaling of parameters. In our experience `drm()` is more robust than is `nls()`; lack of robustness of `nls()` has also been pointed out elsewhere (Nash, 2014).

The estimated variance-covariance of the parameter estimates $(\mathrm{cov}(\hat{\beta}))$ is obtained as the scaled inverse of the observed information matrix, which consists of second-order partial derivatives of f with regard to the model parameters $\beta_1, \ldots, \beta_p$:

$$\mathrm{cov}(\hat{\beta}) = \hat{\sigma}^2 \left(\left\{ \frac{\partial^2 f}{\partial \beta_{p_1} \partial \beta_{p_2}} \right\}_{p_1, p_2 \in \{1, \ldots, p\}} \right)^{-1} = \hat{\sigma}^2 \left(\frac{\partial^2 f}{\partial \beta_{p_1} \partial \beta_{p_2}} \right)^{-1} \quad (A.2)$$

The scaling factor $\hat{\sigma}$ is the residual standard error, which is estimated in the same way as in linear regression. The observed information matrix ("hessian") in equation (A.2) is approximated numerically in `optim()` upon convergence. However, it is not even a requirement that the inverse is available: if it is not then NAs are returned for standard errors.

A.2   Maximum likelihood estimation

In order to obtain parameter estimates, the following expression has to be maximized in terms of β values in order to obtain parameter estimates:

$$\log \text{likelihood} = \sum_{i=1}^{n} l\{y_i, f(x_i, \beta)\} \quad (A.3)$$

where l denotes the logarithm-transformed likelihood function for a single observation (i.e., we look for the β values that render the value of this function as large as possible). The likelihood is entirely defined by the data and the model assumptions, i.e., distributional assumptions and dose-response model function. The log likelihood value for a given dose-response model fit may be obtained using the function `logLik()`.

Estimation based on the maximum likelihood principle provides approximate estimated standard errors and, consequently, approximate confidence intervals. In particular, estimated standard errors are obtained from the estimated variance-covariance matrix of the parameter estimates, which is calculated (approximated numerically) as the inverse of the observed information matrix based on second derivatives of the log likelihood function (van der Vaart, 1998):

$$\mathrm{cov}(\hat{\beta}) = \left(\frac{\partial^2 l}{\partial \beta_{p_1} \partial \beta_{p_2}} \right)^{-1} \quad (A.4)$$

The estimated variance-covariance matrix is available through the function `vcov()`. The estimated standard errors are the square root values of the diagonal elements in this matrix.

Likelihood ratio tests can be used for comparing nested models. Moreover, information criteria such as AIC and BIC can also be calculated and used for comparing non-nested models such as comparing different choices of the model function F.

As detailed below, maximum likelihood estimation is used for fitting dose-response models to binomial, count, and time-to-event data, including models for binomial data where natural immunity and/or natural mortality is present (Finney, 1971).

A.2.1 Binomial dose-response data

A binary response can take on values 0 or 1. A binomial response is the sum of a fixed number of binary responses (the number of 1's). Specifically, let Y_i denote a binomial response obtained in a dose-response experiment while a dose x_i was applied. Then the statistical model may be specified as follows:

$$E(Y_i) = nf(x_i, \beta)$$
$$SD(Y_i) = \sqrt{nf(x_i, \beta)(1 - f(x_i, \beta))} \tag{A.5}$$

Thus, the standard deviation of a binomially distributed response depends solely on the number of basic binary experiments and on the assumed dose-response model function.

A.2.2 Count dose-response data

A.2.2.1 The Poisson distribution

Let Y_i denote the count observed corresponding to the dose x_i. Then the statistical model may be specified as follows:

$$E(Y_i) = f(x_i, \beta)$$
$$SD(Y_i) = \sqrt{f(x_i, \beta)} \tag{A.6}$$

Thus, the standard deviation of a Poisson distributed count is equal to the square root of the mean of the count. For instance, counts with mean 10 will most of the time lie between $10 - 2 \cdot \sqrt{10}$ and $10 + 2 \cdot \sqrt{10}$, that is in the interval $[4, 16]$. Likewise, counts with mean 100 will most of the time lie between $[80, 120]$. Therefore the variation of a Poisson distributed count is somewhat constrained and it will often not suffice to describe the extent of variation observed in reality in count data. Such excess variation compared to the Poisson distribution is usually referred to as over-dispersion (Morgan, 1992, Chapter 6).

Weights may also be incorporated in the Poisson model:

$$E(Y_i) = f(x_i, \beta) \cdot w_i \tag{A.7}$$

where w_i denotes the weight associated with the count Y_i (Delignette-Muller et al., 2014b). As before the standard deviation is equal to the square root of the mean.

A.2.2.2 The negative-binomial distribution

The Poisson model assumes that the standard deviation is equal to the square root of the mean. However, when dealing with count data, it is not unusual to observe larger variation than predicted by the Poisson model. One way to deal with such over-dispersion is to turn to the negative binomial distribution, which has an additional parameter that allows the standard deviation to differ from the square root of the mean. Specifically the negative-binomial distribution implies the following mean and standard deviation:

$$E(Y_i) = f(x_i, \beta)$$
$$SD(Y_i) = \sqrt{f(x_i, \beta) + \omega(x_i, \beta)^2} \qquad \text{(A.8)}$$

where the parameter $\omega \geq 0$ reflects the degree of over-dispersion in the data: the value 0 corresponds to the Poisson model (no overdispersion).

A.2.3 Time-to-event-response data

The statistical model corresponds to assuming that probabilities of an event happening in the different monitoring intervals are described by a multinomial distribution (McCullagh and Nelder, 1989, pp. 164–184, Jager *et al.*, 2011), with probabilities determined by the assumed dose-response model. Specifically, for each monitoring interval $]t_{j-1}, t_j]$ the estimation procedure will seek to match optimally the corresponding observed proportions of events n_j/n against the probabilities of the event happening. More specifically, the likelihood function, which is maximized as a function of the model parameters in order to obtain the parameter estimates, is defined as the product of the probabilities of events happening in the different monitoring intervals, based on all data. In practice, maximization of the logarithm-transformed likelihood, which results in the same estimates, is more computationally convenient:

$$l = \sum_{j=1}^{q} n_j \log(F(t_j) - F(t_{j-1})) \qquad \text{(A.9)}$$

Monitoring intervals where no event was observed may be left out of the analysis as they will not contribute to the estimation ($n_j = 0$ implies a zero term in the log likelihood); in some cases they have to be left out to achieve convergence of the estimation procedure.

The implicit assumption of the above log likelihood is that right-censoring only happens at the end of the experiment, i.e., it is possible to follow all seeds or organisms until the end of the experiment unless the event of interest happens. However, it could also happen that some seeds or organisms are right-censored during the experiment, e.g., seeds are dormant. Thus, the log likelihood would need to be modified slightly (Ritz *et al.*, 2013b).

Model checking can be done by visually assessing the agreement between the observed cumulative germination curve and the fitted curve based on, or by looking at, the residual plot based on cumulative residuals (McCullagh and Nelder, 1989, p. 179).

A.3 The transform-both-sides approach

The transform-both-sides approach implies that both the response and the nonlinear model function are shifted by a constant C and then transformed by a suitable function g_λ (Carroll and Ruppert, 1984). The resulting model for the mean of the transformed response looks like this:

$$E\{g_\lambda(y + C)\} = g_\lambda(f(x, (\beta_1, \ldots, \beta_p)) + C) \qquad (A.10)$$

with the transformed response on the left-hand side and the transformed model function on the right-hand side. Usually the function g_λ is taken to be the Box-Cox transformation $g_\lambda(y) = (y^\lambda - 1)/\lambda$ for some suitable choice of $\lambda \in \mathbb{R}$. The value $\lambda = 1$ implies no transformation whilst $\lambda = 0$ corresponds to the logarithm transformation. All other values of λ correspond to power transformations. It is noteworthy that the Box-Cox transformation may alleviate variance heterogeneity and some skewness in the distribution of the response and thus recover a normal distribution, but it may not remedy other problems with the distributional assumptions such as counts observed with ties (Ritz and Van der Vliet, 2009).

The package *drc* provides a `boxcox` method, which has been implemented in much the same way as the corresponding method for linear models available in the package *MASS* (Venables and Ripley, 2002). There is, however, a choice between a profiling approach as used for linear models in *MASS* or a more robust analysis of variance (ANOVA) approach where the optimal λ is estimated from a more general ANOVA model, i.e., a linear model, and not from the specified dose-response model; the latter requires replicate observations for at least some doses.

Manual specification of the transformation is also possible through the arguments `bcVal` and `bcAdd`, which correspond to λ and C in equation (A.10), respectively. Using a specific transformation (i.e., a specific value of λ and possibly C) based on previous experience should be preferred over using a data-driven choice.

A.4 Robust estimation

One way to handle observations that seem to be extreme or deviating in one way or another as compared to the bulk of the observations is to apply a robust estimation procedure, which will weigh down the influence of such observations.

In *drc* robust dose-response analysis with a continuous response is available through the argument `robust` using the same models as considered in the case of robust linear regression (Venables and Ripley, 2002), except for the model based on Hampel's ψ, which is currently not implemented. However, it may be difficult to fit such robust nonlinear models unless accurate starting values for the model parameters are provided.

The estimated "information"-type variance-covariance has the following form (Huber, 1981; Stromberg, 1993):

$$\text{cov}(\hat{\beta}) = \tilde{\sigma}^2 \left(\frac{\partial^2 \rho}{\partial \beta_{p_1} \partial \beta_{p_2}} \right)^{-1} \tag{A.11}$$

where the function ρ controls the influence of observations on the estimation procedure (e.g., $\rho(y) = y^2$ corresponds to ordinary nonlinear least squares estimation). Once parameter estimates have been obtained, all methods and extractors available in *drc* may be used as if the model fit had been obtained using maximum likelihood estimation.

A.5 Sandwich variance estimators

Consider the situation where a dose-response model has been chosen with mean function f, which is correctly specified, but the assumptions regarding normality and/or the variance homogeneity are not satisfied. In this case, the estimated standard errors from the model assuming normality and variance homogeneity will be inconsistent: They will not approach the true standard errors as the sample size increases. However, even though the model is mis-specified with regard to some of the distributional assumptions, it is still possible to obtain consistent estimates of the standard errors by adjusting the estimated variance-covariance matrix (Carroll and Ruppert, 1988, p. 128).

In case of replicates, one way to calculate robust standard errors is to imagine that the standard error of a predicted response corresponding to a dose included in the experiment is being scaled up or down according to the magnitude of residuals for that particular dose relative to the residual standard error. So there can be different scaling at work for different doses. We give the mathematical definition below.

The modified variance-covariance matrix is defined below.

$$\widehat{\text{var}}(\hat{\beta}) = s^2 \hat{B} \hat{M} \hat{B} \tag{A.12}$$

The matrix $\hat{M}$ is a function of the first derivatives of the log likelihood function and $s^2 \hat{B}$ is the usual variance-covariance matrix. This equation is valid as long as the mean structure is correct and independence can be assumed. Therefore, the resulting estimated variance-covariance matrix is said to be robust against misspecification of the distributional assumptions. If the model is correctly specified, we have the equality $\hat{M} = \hat{B}^{-1}$, and the modified variance-covariance matrix reduces to the usual model-based variance-covariance matrix.

The modified variance-covariance matrix is often called a sandwich variance estimator due to the particular product form on the right-hand side of Equation (A.12). The resulting standard errors are referred to as robust whereas the usual estimated nonrobust variance-covariance matrix results in naïve standard errors. More detailed explanations can be found in White (1981), Carroll and Ruppert (1988, pp. 209–213), White (1996, Chapter 5), and Zeileis (2006).

The use of sandwich variance estimators is attractive because we avoid having to find a transformation or specify a variance model but can still adjust for deviations from the model assumptions. The sandwich variance estimators are obtained in *drc* by utilizing the packages *lmtest* and *sandwich* (Zeileis and Hothorn, 2002; Zeileis, 2006).

A.6 Constrained estimation

By default, unconstrained estimation is carried out by `drm()`, although for most models there are actually constraints on at least some of the model parameters, e.g., ED_{50} needs to be positive. Likewise, there may also be constraints needed to ensure uniqueness of the model fits, e.g., the slope parameter b should be negative for an increasing dose-response relationship to ensure that c is the lower asymptote and d the upper asymptote. In practice, such constraints may often be indirectly enforced through the appropriate choice of starting values.

However, in principle, any of the aforementioned estimation procedures may be combined with the use of constraints where the range of one or more parameters is restricted, e.g., to certain intervals by setting lower and upper bounds (so-called box constraints) that are different from $-\infty$ and ∞, respectively. This is possible with `drm()` using the arguments `lowerl` and `upperl`, which, if specified, will invoke constrained optimization through the method "L-BFGS-B" in `optim()`.

A.7 Two-stage estimation for hierarchical models

Estimating the unknown parameters in the hierarchical nonlinear model by maximum likelihood is a challenge, as the likelihood function includes an improper integral, that is, does not have a closed-form solution (Demidenko,

2013). Several estimators for β are available, where the most popular among R users utilizes the Lindstrom-Bates algorithm.

A.7.1 Technical replicates

If there is large uncertainty about each observation for an individual, e.g., using a device that exhibits large variability for each measurement, this additional source of variance can be represented by observing multiple technical replicates from the same experimental unit. A simple two-stage analysis strategy can be applied, calculating an average response for each individual and assuming a dose-response model for the estimated averages in a second stage. It is obvious that this approach only works for repeated measurements at a single dose level within an individual. As the uncertainty about estimating each average is ignored in the second stage, there is some loss of information as each average obtains the same weight. Hence, the same number of observations is required for each individual.

A.7.2 Two-stage approaches

If an experimental design is planned with repeated measurements for different dose levels within an individual, the two-stage approach for the technical replicates can be extended to a more general framework (Demidenko, 2013).

1. In a first step, a separate curve $f_j\left(x_j, \beta_j\right)$ is fitted for each of the M individuals, using nonlinear least-squares. For each of the M models we obtain a set of coefficient estimates $\hat{\beta}_j$ together with the corresponding variance estimates.

2. Estimates for the population parameters can be obtained in a second step, treating the estimated coefficients for each individual as a new response in a linear model.

$$\beta_j \approx A_j\tilde{\beta} + B_j b_j + \epsilon_j^\star$$

The first stage requires that each individual curve can be fitted; that is, the number of observations need to be larger than the number of unknown parameters and the full dose range should be covered. Further, it requires that there is no common parameter shared between individual curves; otherwise, it would not be possible to fit the curves separately from each other in the first stage.

For the estimation of the population parameters in the second step, a method-of-moments estimator of the between-individual variance Ψ can be obtained, followed by a generalized least-squares estimation of $\tilde{\beta}$ (Demidenko, 2013). Alternatively, $\tilde{\beta}$ and Ψ can be estimated by maximum likelihood (Davidian and Giltinan, 1995, Chapter 5.3), incorporating the uncertainty about estimating the individual $\hat{\beta}_j$ by a residual term $\epsilon_j^\star$. The individual residual variances are fixed during the maximization of the likelihood in the second step.

The concept of the two-stage approach can also be presented as a meta-analysis framework (Jiang and Kopp-Schneider, 2014; Viechtbauer, 2010). Assuming that the individual curves originate from separate experiments, one can combine the estimated coefficients by a weighted average. The weights depend on the residual variance of the individual curves and the between-experiment variance. Again, several methods of moments and maximum likelihood estimators are available to obtain the heterogeneity estimators (Kalaian and Raudenbush, 1996; Berkey *et al.*, 1998; van Houwelingen *et al.*, 2002).

A.7.3   Lindstrom-Bates algorithm

The Lindstrom-Bates algorithm is a two-stage procedure, approximating the nonlinear model by a linear mixed-effects model (Lindstrom and Bates, 1990; Pinheiro and Bates, 2000).

1. In the first step, a penalized least-squares algorithm is applied, minimizing

$$\sum_{j=1}^{M} \|\boldsymbol{y}_j - \boldsymbol{f}_j\left(\boldsymbol{x}_j, \boldsymbol{\beta}_j\right)\|^2 + \|\boldsymbol{\Delta} \boldsymbol{b}_j\|^2$$

   to find estimates of the fixed-effects parameters while holding the precision factor $\boldsymbol{\Delta}$ fixed, which factors the precision matrix of the random effects and expresses it relative to the precision of the residuals.

2. In the second step, a linear mixed-effects model is applied to a vector of weights as a new response and design matrices $\hat{\boldsymbol{X}}_j$ and $\hat{\boldsymbol{Z}}_j$ for the fixed and random effects, which are obtained at the parameter estimates from the first step by

$$\hat{w}_j = \boldsymbol{y}_j - \boldsymbol{f}_j\left(\boldsymbol{x}_j, \hat{\boldsymbol{\beta}}_j\right) + \hat{\boldsymbol{X}}_j \hat{\tilde{\boldsymbol{\beta}}} + \hat{\boldsymbol{Z}}_j \hat{\boldsymbol{b}}_j$$

$$\hat{\boldsymbol{X}}_j = \left.\frac{\partial \boldsymbol{f}_j}{\partial \tilde{\boldsymbol{\beta}}'}\right|_{\hat{\tilde{\boldsymbol{\beta}}}, \hat{\boldsymbol{b}}_j}, \qquad \hat{\boldsymbol{Z}}_j = \left.\frac{\partial \boldsymbol{f}_j}{\partial \boldsymbol{b}_j'}\right|_{\hat{\tilde{\boldsymbol{\beta}}}, \hat{\boldsymbol{b}}_j}$$

The precision factor $\boldsymbol{\Delta}$ that is estimated in the second step is again plugged in the penalized least-squares step. The algorithm then iterates between the two steps until convergence. Pinheiro and Bates (2000) and Demidenko (2013) provide additional information about the algorithm and numerical details of its implementation in R.

Following Pinheiro and Bates (2000), we can assume the following distribution for the fixed-effects estimator:

$$\hat{\tilde{\boldsymbol{\beta}}} \sim N\left(\tilde{\boldsymbol{\beta}}, \sigma^2 \left[\sum_{j=1}^{M} \hat{\boldsymbol{X}}_j \boldsymbol{\Sigma}_j^{-1} \hat{\boldsymbol{X}}_j\right]^{-1}\right), \quad \text{where} \quad \boldsymbol{\Sigma}_j = \boldsymbol{I} - \hat{\boldsymbol{Z}}_j \boldsymbol{\Delta}^{-1} \boldsymbol{\Delta}^{-T} \hat{\boldsymbol{Z}}_j^T$$

A.8   Starting values and self-starter functions

Due to the nonlinearity of most dose-response models, a critically important aspect of estimation in dose-response analysis is the choice of the so-called starting values for the model parameters. The numerical optimization procedure used for estimating the model parameters needs to be initialized at some values of the model parameters from which it can iteratively approach the optimal values as judged by some criterion. The optimal values of the model parameters are the parameter estimates, which we interpret as providing the best-fitting dose-response curve(s) to the data.

Although the starting values may be derived from the same dose-response data for which a dose-response model has to be fitted, the starting values are not to be understood as parameter estimates and they cannot be used for drawing any kind of statistical inference. They are simply a tool for getting the estimation to work.

The estimation procedures used for dose-response analysis in this book are iterative and they need to be initiated by starting values for the model parameters. The choice of starting values may crucially affect whether convergence is eventually achieved. Thus, availability of good starting values facilitates parameter estimation in nonlinear models.

Starting values may be obtained either by using parameter estimates previously reported for similar experiments or, in a data-driven way, by using the dose-response data themselves to elicit relevant information. For instance, within weed science, routine calculation of starting values for log-logistic models from simple linear regression models of transformed responses dates back at least to Streibig *et al.* (1993), utilizing extended linearization techniques previously used for probit analysis and modified for nonlinear regression (Streibig, 1981). The flexibility of **R** has made it possible to implement so-called self-starter functions that return data-driven starting values for the model parameters. In **R**, self-starter functions are available for the function nls(). In *drc* the above-mentioned data-driven linearization technique has been extended to other types of dose-response models and it is now available for all built-in *drc* models. Use of the self-starter function is the default setting, which may, however, be overruled by supplying starting values manually through the argument start. The function getInitial() may be used to obtain the starting values that were actually used for obtaining a particular model fit.

If a dose-response model is fitted to dose-response data with multiple curves, then starting values are needed for all model parameters in all groups. The parameters should be provided for each model parameter, i.e., the values for the parameter b first, next the one for the parameter c, and so on in alphabetic order.

More sophisticated self-starter functions have been proposed (Normolle, 1993), but so far they have not been implemented in *drc* except for log-logistic models.

A.9 Confidence intervals

For a dose-response model that assumes normally distributed response values, the confidence interval of a parameter is defined as the corresponding parameter estimate $\pm$ K $\cdot$ estimated standard error of the parameter estimate. To obtain a 95% confidence interval, the constant K is equal to the 97.5% percentile in a t distribution with degrees of freedom equal to the number of response values minus the number of parameters in the model function used in the model.

For all other types of dose-response data, Wald-type confidence intervals are used, i.e., to obtain a 95% confidence interval, the constant K is equal to the 97.5% percentile in the standard normal distribution ($K = 1.96$). These intervals are often referred to as Wald intervals.

By definition, these confidence intervals are symmetric around the estimate, which occasionally may result in lower bounds that are unrealistic, e.g., a negative lower limit for the confidence interval for $ED50$ or for the confidence band for the entire dose-response curve. There are several ways to ensure that they fall within a realistic range. One simple approach is to truncate lower limits and bounds at 0 (Feng and McCulloch, 1992); this approach is implemented in the predict() method.

A pointwise confidence band for the dose-response curve is a collection of confidence intervals corresponding to doses in a given interval. The band is pointwise as 95% coverage is only established for each confidence interval, but not for the entire confidence band, which will have somewhat less than 95% coverage.

Inverse regression of the confidence band of the dose-response function also leads to asymmetric confidence intervals for ED values (Nottingham and Birch, 2000). For ED values too close to 0 or 1 the resulting confidence intervals may degenerate, having either 0 as the lower limit or ∞ as the upper limit.

A.10 Prediction and inverse regression

There are a number of functions available in *drc* for obtaining predicted values from a dose-response model fit. Notably, there are the general-purpose methods fitted() and predict(). The latter may also provide confidence or prediction intervals (controlled through the argument type). The function backfit() may be used for obtaining the estimated doses that correspond to the observed average response at each dose.

Estimating doses corresponding to specific response levels is often of particular interest in dose-response analysis. Such estimates are obtained by solving an inverse regression problem, which may be approached either by means of after-fitting or using a re-parameterization. After-fitting means solving the inverse regression problem *after* having fitted the model. For some models the solution may be derived explicitly (e.g., log-logistic models (Streibig and Jensen, 2000; Ritz and Streibig, 2005)) whereas for other models only numerical solutions are available, e.g., hormesis models (Cedergreen *et al.*, 2005). Re-parameterization means fitting the model again using a reparameterized model function where the parameter of interest is a model parameter.

After-fitting relies on the so-called delta method, which is a statistical method for obtaining approximate standard errors for derived parameter estimates, i.e., parameter estimates that are functions or transformations of the estimated model parameters. The intuitive explanation is as follows: For a specific function $g(\beta)$ of the model parameter β, the delta method utilizes mathematical calculus (first-order differentiation of g in β) to derive a scaling factor that will convert the estimated standard error of $\hat{\beta}$ into an estimated approximate standard error of the derived parameter estimate $g(\hat{\beta})$. It works if it is reasonable to assume local linearity of the function g in the neighbourhood of $\hat{\beta}$; it can be a nonlinear function, but it should not fluctuate too rapidly. For a more detailed and technical explanation, we refer to Weisberg (2005).

A practical implication of the after-fitting approach is that it suffices to fit a dose-response model once, in a parameterization that has proven to be the most stable for estimation. In our opinion, after-fitting provides a major improvement over the often quite unstable re-parameterization approach.

A.10.1 Effective dose

The most prominent example of a derived parameter obtained using inverse regression is the dose that results in a halfway reduction between the lower and upper limits of the dose-response curve f as doses approach infinity and 0, respectively. This parameter is often denoted $ED50$ or $EC50$ for continuous responses, and $LD50$ or $LC50$ for binomial responses, and t_{50} for event-time responses.

For a monotonously decreasing mean function f, the effective dose for $0 < \alpha < 1$ ($ED100\alpha$) is defined as the solution to the following equation:

$$f(ED100\alpha, \beta) = (1 - \alpha) \lim_{x \to 0} f(x, \beta) + \alpha \lim_{x \to \infty} f(x, \beta) = (1 - \alpha)c + \alpha d \quad \text{(A.13)}$$

Note that these limits are well defined and finite for dose-response models (for most models in *drc* they correspond to the parameters d and c, respectively). For a monotonously increasing mean function the same equation is obtained by interchanging the limits.

The resulting effective dose is a relative quantity, defined in terms of a percentage reduction. For instance, $ED50$ ($\alpha = 0.50$) is the dose resulting in a 50% reduction in the average response relative to the lower and upper limits of f. Such relative effective doses are mostly suitable for continuous responses. For increasing α, the corresponding $ED100\alpha$ will be increasing as a consequence of f being a decreasing function.

For binomial responses, absolute effective doses referring to the entire probability scale $[0, 1]$, which do not necessarily coincide with the lower and upper limits of the estimated dose-response curve, are usually more relevant. In general, an absolute effective dose EDy_0 corresponding to an average response y_0 may be defined as the solution to the following equation:

$$f(EDy_0, \beta) = y_0 \tag{A.14}$$

An absolute effective dose for $y_0 \in]c, d[$ may always be calculated as some relative effective dose for a suitably derived α value. In some cases, this approach will involve parameter estimates of the lower and upper limits, but at present the variation in these estimates will not be propagated to the estimated effective dose.

Estimated effective doses are obtained by inserting parameter estimates and solving equation (A.13) with regards to the derived parameter $ED100\alpha$. In *drc*, the function ED() will calculate estimated effective doses, and the argument type controls the type of effective dose being calculated: relative (default) or absolute. Note also that for hormesis models, effective doses may also be meaningfully defined for some $\alpha < 0$ (by setting the argument bound=TRUE in ED()). Model-averaged estimated ED values may be obtained through the function maED() (Kang *et al.*, 2000).

A.10.2   Relative potency

The ratio of two effective doses $ED100\alpha_1$ and $ED100\alpha_2$ ($0 < \alpha_1 < 1$ and $0 < \alpha_2 < 1$) of two fitted dose-response curves denoted A and B, say, is defined as follows:

$$\rho(\alpha_1, \alpha_2) = \frac{ED_A 100\alpha_1}{ED_B 100\alpha_2}, \qquad 0 < \alpha_1, \alpha_2 < 1$$

For the important special case where $\alpha_1 = \alpha_2$, the ratio is referred to as the relative potency (Finney, 1971), and it is interpreted as a measure for quantifying the strength of one substance over another, i.e., a pairwise comparison based on a ratio. The term selectivity index is also sometimes used (Christensen *et al.*, 2003). In general, the ratio may be interpreted as the order of magnitude of the window between harmful and safe for appropriate choices of α_1 and α_2, e.g., 0.1 and 0.9. In some special cases ("parallelism") the relative potency is constant between two dose-response curves for all values satisfying $\alpha_1 = \alpha_2$. More often it will change with the value of $\alpha_1 = \alpha_2$ and this can be investigated using the function relpot() (Ritz *et al.*, 2006).

In *drc* the extractor function EDcomp() may be used to obtain estimated relative potencies or differences between effective doses. By default the corresponding standard errors are derived using the delta method and confidence intervals are based on these standard errors (indicated through the argument interval = "delta") in combination with the t- or z-value (a percentile in an appropriate t- or normal distribution). Alternatively, confidence intervals based on the approach of Fieller may be used (interval = "fieller") (Morgan, 1992; Faraggi *et al.*, 2003). For the special case of the log-logistic model where $log(ED_{50})$ is a model parameter ($\tilde{e}$), confidence intervals on the original dose scale may be retrieved through back transformation (interval = "fls").

Appendix B

Dose-response model functions

In this chapter, we provide detailed descriptions of dose-response models belonging to four main classes of models: log-logistic, log-normal, Weibull type 1, and Weibull type 2 models. These four classes of models may be seen as direct extensions of the four types of generalized linear models proposed by McCullagh and Nelder (1989, pp. 108–109) for analysis of binomial data, corresponding to the logit, probit, log-log, and complementary log-log link functions, respectively. The extensions include more model parameters and are useful for various types of dose-response data, not only binomial dose-response data. Some other types of dose-response models are also introduced. Table B.1 and Table B.2 provide an overview of the models available in *drc*. However, this chapter does not provide an exhaustive account of all available dose-response models.

Many of these dose-response model functions, which we describe below, may be constructed via a cumulative distribution function (cdf) or some other suitable function F, say, in the following way:

$$f(x) = c + (d - c)F(x, b, \ldots) \tag{B.1}$$

(Seber and Wild, 1989, p. 337). The parameter c denotes the lower asymptote or limit of the dose-response model, and the parameter d denotes the upper asymptote or horizontal limit of the dose-response curve. There will always be a parameter b, which, in one way or another, will reflect the rate of change of the dose-response curve between the upper and lower limits, analogous with the slope coefficient of a simple linear regression model. However, in general, dose-response models have no equivalent to an intercept and hence there is no model parameter named a. The number of additional parameters (denoted $\ldots$) will depend on the choice of F (usually 1–3) and these parameters will be denoted e, f etc.

In addition, many of the model functions are scale invariant in the sense that the model itself, usually through the parameter e, which acts as a scaling factor, accommodates the magnitude of doses. Likewise, many of the model functions involve the logarithm. We use the natural logarithm and its inverse, the exponential function (power of e), but most models may also be formulated using any other logarithm (resulting in a slightly different reparameterization of the models). For instance, models using the base-10 logarithm are occasionally used.

B.1   Log-logistic models

The log-logistic models are by far the most commonly used dose-response models (e.g., Environment Canada, 2005; Van der Vliet and Ritz, 2013). The basic model may be derived from the cdf of the standard log-logistic distribution.

Sometimes log-logistic models are confusingly called logistic models (e.g., Ritz and Streibig, 2005). Strictly speaking, logistic models, however, constitute a different class of models and are in general not as suitable for describing dose-response data as they are defined for the entire real axis and not only for the non-negative dose scale (Ritz, 2010). Logistic models may, however, be useful in other contexts where the x axis is not confined to the non-negative part.

B.1.1   Four-parameter log-logistic models

The four-parameter log-logistic model corresponds to the following model function:

$$f(x, (b, c, d, e)) = c + \frac{d - c}{1 + \exp(b(\log(x) - \log(e)))}$$

$$= c + \frac{d - c}{1 + (x/e)^b} = c + (d - c)(1 + (x/e)^b)^{-1} \qquad (B.2)$$

The four parameters are b, c, d, and e. The parameter e, which by definition has to be positive, corresponds to the dose producing a response half-way between the upper limit d and lower limit c, i.e., the parameter e is the ED50. The slope parameter b reflects the steepness of the dose-response curve at the dose ED50. Specifically, the relative slope of the log-logistic model function has the opposite sign as compared to the sign of the parameter b. This is a consequence of the parameterization used in *drc*, a choice rooted in the standard terminology used in weed science. The actual slope of the tangent of the log-logistic model function at e is equal to:

$$\frac{-b}{(d - c)/(4e)} \qquad (B.3)$$

So, apart from the sign, there is a scaling factor, depending on c, d, and e, that converts the parameter b into the slope; therefore, the use of the phrase "relative slope." Note that the scaling factor may be viewed as a kind of normalization factor involving the range of the response. As a consequence, estimated b values often lie in the range 0.5 to 20 in absolute value, in a way centered around 1, regardless of the assay or experiment generating the data.

The four-parameter log-logistic model may also be parameterized in other ways than shown in Eq. (B.2). One such alternative parameterization is where the logarithm of $ED50$ denoted by $\tilde{e}$, say, is a model parameter instead of e

as in the following equation (B.4):

$$f(x, (b, c, d, \tilde{e})) = c + \frac{d - c}{1 + \exp(b(\log(x) - \tilde{e}))} \tag{B.4}$$

This second version of the four-parameter log-logistic model may be preferred for dose-response analysis involving very small datasets (<15–20) where a normally distributed parameter estimate may more reasonably be assumed on a logarithm-transformed dose scale than the original dose scale.

The four-parameter log-logistic model is also sometimes referred to as the (sigmoidal) E-max model (MacDougall, 2006) or Hill model, and the slope parameter b is also sometimes referred to as the Hill coefficient or factor.

B.1.1.1 Three-parameter version

In the three-parameter log-logistic model function, the parameter c is fixed at the value 0:

$$f(x, (b, d, e)) = \frac{d}{1 + \exp(b(\log(x) - \log(e)))} \tag{B.5}$$

This model function may be helpful in case there are no data to properly estimate the lower limit. This assumption should ideally also be reasoned on biological or toxicological grounds.

B.1.1.2 Two-parameter version

If the parameters c and d are fixed at 0 and 1, respectively, then the so-called two-parameter log-logistic model is obtained:

$$f(x, (b, e)) = \frac{1}{1 + \exp(b(\log(x) - \log(e)))} = \frac{\exp(-b(\log(x) - \log(e)))}{1 + \exp(-b(\log(x) - \log(e)))} \tag{B.6}$$

The rightmost formula shows that, for binomial data, the two-parameter log-logistic model is equivalent to the logistic regression model with $\log(x)$ as the only explanatory variable (in a slightly different parameterization than the ordinary logistic regression model).

B.1.1.3 E-max and Michaelis-Menten models

Another special case is the Michaelis-Menten model. The standard two-parameter Michaelis-Menten model is obtained by putting $b = 1$ and $c = 0$ in Equation (B.2):

$$f(x, (d, e)) = \frac{dx}{x + e} \tag{B.7}$$

In a medical or pharmaceutical context, this model is usually called the (hyperbolic) E-max model (MacDougall, 2006). It is also sometimes referred to as the rectangular hyperbola model.

The three-parameter shifted Michaelis-Menten model is defined as follows:

$$f(x, (c, d, e)) = c + \frac{d - c}{1 + (e/x)} = c + \frac{(d - c)x}{x + e} \qquad (B.8)$$

Michaelis-Menten models are some of the best-known models of enzyme kinetics but they can also model numerous other biological relationships (e.g., Ritz and Streibig, 2008, pp. 2–3).

B.1.2   Extensions

B.1.2.1   Generalized log-logistic models

Generalized log-logistic model functions may be obtained based on cdf's of the Burr type III and XII distributions (Pant and Headrick, 2013). These functions involve one additional asymmetry parameter compared to the four-parameter log-logistic model and they include the four-parameter log-logistic model as a special case. Inclusion of the parameter f implies that the parameter e loses its interpretation as ED50, although ED50 may still be estimated as a derived parameter.

The five-parameter Burr type III generalized log-logistic model function was proposed by Finney (1979) for describing continuous dose-response data. It is also known as the Richards model (Seber and Wild, 1989, pp. 332–333, Sand *et al.*, 2006). Specifically, the model function is defined as follows:

$$\begin{aligned} f(x, (b, c, d, e, f)) &= c + \frac{d - c}{(1 + \exp[b\{\log(x) - \log(e)\}])^f} \\ &= c + (d - c)(1 + (x/e)^b)^{-f} \end{aligned} \qquad (B.9)$$

where the parameter f, which should be positive, controls the degree of asymmetry: $f < 1$ and $f > 1$ lead to a more rapid or a slower descent towards the limits (for a more detailed explanation, see below under Weibull models); see Sand *et al.* (2006) for an illustration of the different types of asymmetry. For $f = 1$ the four-parameter log-logistic model is recovered, i.e., there is no asymmetry. Gottschalk and Dunn (2005) provide a more detailed description of the asymmetry.

For binomial data, the special case of the Burr type III generalized log-logistic model obtained by fixing the lower and upper limits at 0 and 1, respectively, is the so-called convenient three-parameter model proposed by Prentice (1976); see also Shao (2000); Scholze *et al.* (2001).

The five-parameter Burr type XII generalized log-logistic model is defined as follows:

$$f(x, (b, c, d, e, f)) = c + (d - c)(1 - (1 + (x/e)^b)^{-f}) \qquad (B.10)$$

This five-parameter model does not seem to have been used in practice for fitting dose-response data. Currently, this model is not in *drc*.

For binomial data there are a number of special cases: the three-parameter model obtained by fixing the lower and upper limits at 0 and 1 (Prentice, 1976; Stukel, 1988), in another parameterization the related three-parameter Aranda-Ordaz model (Aranda-Ordaz, 1981), and the so-called approximate beta-Poisson model for $b = 1$, $c = 0$, and $d = 1$ (e.g., Namata *et al.*, 2008).

B.1.2.2 A model with two slope parameters

The five-parameter baroflex model is a modification of the four-parameter log-logistic model to include two slope parameters. It was originally proposed by Ricketts and Head (1999) for studying baroreflex properties in humans. It was proposed as an extension of the four-parameter logistic model. However, a similar extension is possible for the four-parameter log-logistic model, making the model more suited for describing dose-response data; this version is implemented in *drc*. The model function is defined as follows:

$$f(x, (b_1, b_2, c, d, e))$$
$$= d + \frac{(d - c)}{1 + g(x) \exp[b_1\{\log(x) - \log(e)\}] + (1 - g(x)) \exp[b_2\{\log(x) - \log(e)\}]}$$
(B.11)

where the helper function g is itself a two-parameter log-logistic function:

$$g(x) = \frac{1}{1 + \exp[k\{\log(x) - \log(e)\}]}$$

with slope parameter defined as $k = 2b_1 b_2 / |b_1 + b_2|$ ($|\cdot|$ denotes absolute value).

B.1.2.3 Hormesis models

Two non-monotonous five-parameter hormesis models, which are derived from the four-parameter log-logistic model, have been proposed by Brain and Cousens (1989) and Cedergreen *et al.* (2005).

The Brain-Cousens model is defined as follows:

$$f(x, (b, c, d, e, f)) = c + \frac{d - c + fx}{1 + (x/e)^b}$$
(B.12)

where the parameter $f \geq 0$ reflects the degree of hormesis, with $f = 0$ implying no hormetic effect as the four-parameter log-logistic model is recovered (Equation (B.2)).

The Cedergreen-Ritz-Streibig model is defined in a similar way, but with an exponential term instead of a linear term in the numerator:

$$f(x, (b, c, d, e, f)) = c + \frac{d - c + f \exp(-1/x^\alpha)}{1 + (x/e)^b}$$
(B.13)

where the parameter f has the same interpretation as in the Brain-Cousens model (Cedergreen *et al.*, 2005). The additional parameter α is usually fixed at a value larger than 0 and less than or equal to 1. The closer α is to 1 the steeper the ascent is towards the hormesis peak.

In contrast to the other log-logistic type models, the Brain-Cousens and Cedergreen-Ritz-Streibig models are sensitive to the magnitudes of the doses, which may need to be manually up- or downscaled appropriately prior to model fitting (Belz and Piepho, 2012).

Moreover, these models can only describe decreasing trends, i.e., they are suitable for modeling so-called inverse j-shaped hormesis models. However, a modified Cedergreen-Ritz-Streibig model functions for u-shaped hormesis models for describing increasing dose-response trends are also available:

$$f(x, (b, c, d, e, f)) = d - \frac{d - c + f \exp(-1/x^\alpha)}{1 + (x/e)^b} \qquad \text{(B.14)}$$

We refer to Garnier-Laplace *et al.* (2010) for an application.

B.1.2.4 Two- and three-phase models

The four-parameter log-logistic model may be seen as a one-phase model reflecting that the response of a single biological mechanism was observed over the dose range. In some cases, multiple mechanisms may be at work and more complex models may be justified.

The two-phase log-logistic model is defined as follows:

$$f(x, (b_1, b_2, c_1, d_1, d_2, e_1, e_2)) = c_1 + \frac{d_1 - c_1}{1 + (x/e_1)^{b_1}} + \frac{d_2}{1 + (x/e_2)^{b_2}} \qquad \text{(B.15)}$$

It is a model with 7 parameters where b_1, c_1, d_1, and e_1 describe the first phase and b_2, d_2, and e_2 describe the second phase, which takes over once the first phase has reached an average response equal to d_1.

The three-phase model is defined similarly but with an additional term. These models are extremely flexible and as a result the model fits may not always look like expected, Therefore, these models are suitable for dose-response data where a two-phase trend is expected and where there are enough data (e.g., Cornou *et al.*, 2013).

B.1.2.5 Fractional polynomial models

For a binomial response, Namata *et al.* (2008) introduced fractional polynomial log-logistic models. These models may be extended in a straightforward way to four-parameter versions that are also suitable for describing continuous dose-response data. The four-parameter model function is defined as follows:

$$f(x, (b, c, d, e)) = c + \frac{d - c}{1 + \exp(b(\log(x + 1))^{p_1} + e(\log(x + 1))^{p_2})}$$

The powers p_1 and p_2 need to be specified in advance (they are not estimated from the data) and p_1 has to be negative, whereas p_2 has to be positive. Following the recommendations of Royston and Altman (1994) the powers should be chosen among the numbers –2, –1, –0.5, 0, 0.5, 1, 2, 3, e.g., some choices are (–0.5, 0.5), (–1,1), (–1,2), (–1,3), or (–2,3).

Fractional polynomial models have been proposed as a flexible class of candidate models for model averaging by including several choices of (p_1, p_2) (Faes *et al.*, 2007; Namata *et al.*, 2008).

Finally, we note that fractional polynomial models may also be derived for log-normal and Weibull models (Namata *et al.*, 2008).

B.2 Log-normal models

Bruce and Versteeg (1992) introduced the four-parameter log-normal dose-response model. We define this model using a slightly different parameterization (following the same conventions as for log-logistic models):

$$f\bigl(x,(b,c,d,e)\bigr) = c + (d-c)\Phi[b\{\log(x) - \log(e)\}] \qquad (B.16)$$

where Φ is the cumulative distribution function of the standard normal distribution. The parameters b, c, d, and e have the same interpretation as in the four-parameter logistic model. Note that the parameter e has to be positive. In particular, the parameter e corresponds to ED50. Three- and two-parameter log-normal models may be defined in the same way as log-logistic models.

The three-parameter model was used by van der Hoeven (1997). Otherwise, log-normal dose-responses for continuous endpoints do not appear to be used often in practice. One reason may be that, in most statistical software packages, they are not readily available in the general formulation given in Equation (B.16). Moreover, as Bruce and Versteeg (1992) noted, the results from log-normal and log-logistic models are almost identical, just like results from logistic regression models with logit and probit link functions are very similar (McCullagh and Nelder, 1989, p. 109).

For binomial data, the two-parameter log-normal model corresponds to the logistic regression model with probit link function and logarithm-transformed dose as only explanatory variable; this model is also referred to as the log-probit model (Sand *et al.*, 2008).

For binomial data, the probit model has been used for a long time (Finney, 1971, Chapter 2). A recent application was reported by Wheeler *et al.* (2006).

B.3   Weibull models

There are two types of Weibull models, Weibull type 1 and Weibull type 2 models. They are constructed in the same way as the Burr type III and XII generalized log-logistic models from a suitable cdf. Sometimes the Weibull models are confused with the Gompertz models, which constitute a different class of models that are generally not suitable for describing dose-response data (Ritz, 2010).

B.3.1   Weibull type 1 models

The four-parameter Weibull type 1 model is defined by the model function:

$$f\{x, (b, c, d, e)\} = c + (d - c)\exp(-\exp[b\{\log(x) - \log(e)\}])$$
$$= c + (d - c)\exp\left(-(x/e)^b\right) \qquad (B.17)$$

where the only restriction on the parameters is that the parameter e has to be positive.

This is the Weibull growth model considered by Piegorsch and Bailer (2005, pp. 79–82) (in a slightly different parameterization). In contrast to the log-logistic model, the parameter e is not equal to ED50, but it is still the location of the inflection point of the dose-response curve. The parameter b is reflecting the steepness of the dose-response curve, being proportional to the slope at the dose equal to e: the larger absolute values the steeper the curve. The asymmetry can be characterized by comparison to the symmetric log-logistic model. The dose-response curve descends slowly from the upper limit, but the curve approaches the lower limit rapidly. In fact, the behaviour of the Weibull type 1 model at the upper limit is very similar to the behaviour of the log-logistic model (which can be seen by using the approximation $\exp u \approx 1 + u$ for u close to 0). The figure shown by McCullagh and Nelder (1989, p. 109) is insightful in order to understand the differences between the four classes of models.

B.3.1.1   Exponential decay model

A special case of the Weibull type 1 model is the exponential decay model with a non-zero lower limit:

$$f(x, (c, d, e)) = c + (d - c)\exp(-x/e) \qquad (B.18)$$

(obtained by fixing b at 1 in the four-parameter Weibull type 1 model). Note that by definition the parameter e is positive, ensuring that the model function is decreasing.

In decay studies, a positive lower limit c could be justified when there are systematic errors in the measurements of the residual concentration of a compound in a medium, or if the degradation becomes very slow due to lack of substrate. The exponential model with lower limit at 0 ($c = 0$) is used by Stephenson *et al.* (2000) (in a slightly different parameterization) for analysis of soil toxicity test data.

B.3.1.2   Other special cases

All models described by Slob (2002) are Weibull type 1 models in the sense that they correspond to the Weibull type 1 model given by Equation (B.17) or a special case derived from Equation (B.17) by fixing one or more parameters at specific values. However, the parameterizations differ slightly.

A special case of the Weibull type 1 when fixing $c = 0$ and $d = 1$ could be useful to describe quantal dose-response data, but it has not been used in practice by ecotoxicologists. This is not entirely surprising as the corresponding generalized linear model with log-log link function for binomial data is also rare (McCullagh and Nelder, 1989, p. 108).

B.3.2   Weibull type 2 models

The second class of Weibull models is defined by the following model function:

$$f\{x, (b, c, d, e)\} = c + (d - c)\{1 - \exp(-\exp[b\{\log(x) - \log(e)\}])\}$$
$$= c + (d - c)\{1 - \exp(-(x/e)^b)\} \qquad (B.19)$$

where again the parameter e has to be positive. The parameter b has the same interpretation as for the Weibull type 1 models.

The Weibull type 2 model differs from the Weibull type 1 model as it exhibits a different form of asymmetry with a rapid change or descent from the upper limit, but a slow approach towards the lower limit. Thus the Weibull type 2 model is different from the log-logistic model close to the upper asymptote (low doses for decreasing data), but very similar to the log-logistic model close to the lower asymptote (McCullagh and Nelder, 1989, p. 109).

B.3.2.1   Asymptotic regression

The asymptotic regression model is a dose-response model that is obtained by setting $b = 1$ in Eq. (B.19):

$$f(x, (c, d, e)) = c + (d - c)(1 - \exp(-x/e)) \qquad (B.20)$$

This model may be seen as an asymmetric alternative to the Michaelis-Menten model for dose-response data with increasing trend (Keller *et al.*, 2002). Asymptotic regression has also been used in animal science to describe weight increase as a function of supplementation dose levels (Kratzer and Littell, 2004).

B.3.2.2 Other special cases

The special case with $c = 0$ is sometimes called the Douglas model in pharmacology (Keller *et al.*, 2002). Caux and Moore (1997) consider the case with the constraints $c = 0$ and $d = 100$. By fixing d at 1 we obtain the first-order multistage model (Downs, 1992; Piegorsch and Bailer, 2005, p. 181); these models are mostly suitable for binomial data. Likewise, the special case obtained for $c = 0$ and $d = 1$ is useful for binomial data, (e.g., Meister and van den Brink, 2000; Scholze *et al.*, 2001). Sometimes this special case is referred to as the extreme value model (e.g., Namata *et al.*, 2008). In another parameterization this model is the well-known generalized linear model with the complementary log-log link function for binomial data (McCullagh and Nelder, 1989, Chapter 4). Finally, the special case obtained by fixing the three parameters c, d, and e at the values 0, 1, and 1, respectively, is the one-hit model described by Edler and Kopp-Schneider (1998).

B.3.2.3 Generalized Weibull-2 model

The four-parameter Weibull-2 model function may be augmented with a fifth parameter, an additional asymmetry parameter f, in the following way:

$$f\{x, (b, c, d, e, f)\} = c + (d - c)\{1 - \exp(-\exp[b\{\log(x) - \log(e)\}])\}^f$$
$$= c + (d - c)\{1 - \exp(-(x/e)^b)\}^f \qquad (B.21)$$

To our knowledge this five-parameter model function has not been used much for fitting dose-response data except for the special case with $b = 1$, which is the so-called Hodgkin-Huxley model (Keller *et al.*, 2002). This model is not in *drc*.

B.4 Other types of models

B.4.1 Gamma models

The four-parameter gamma model is defined using this function:

$$f(x, (b, c, d, e)) = c + (d - c)\Gamma(bx, e, 1)$$

where Γ denotes the distribution function for a Γ distribution with shape parameter e and scale parameter 1 (Wheeler and Bailer, 2009).

B.4.2 Multistage models

The four-parameter multistage model of second order is an extension of the exponential decay model where dose squared now also enters the exponent:

$$f(x, c(b_1, b_2, c, d)) = c + (d - c)\exp(-b_1 x - b_2 x^2)$$

The parameters b_1 and b_2 have to be non-negative to ensure a decreasing dose-response model function (Piegorsch and Bailer, 2005, p. 181). In principle higher-order terms could be included in the exponent, but they may hardly be needed in practice. The quantal-linear and quantal-quadratic models for binomial data are obtained by setting $c = 0$, $d = 1$, and either $b_2 = 0$ or $b_1 = 0$ (Wheeler and Bailer, 2009). The exponential decay model defined in Equation (B.18) is a special case, which is sometimes referred to as a one-stage model (Fang *et al.*, 2015).

B.4.3 NEC

Another built-in model is the so-called "no effect concentration" (NEC) model proposed by Pires *et al.* (2002). The corresponding model function involves four parameters:

$$f(x, (b, c, d, e)) = \begin{cases} c + (d - c)\exp(b(x - e)) & \text{if } x > e \\ d & \text{if } x \le e \end{cases}$$

This model is a so-called threshold model such that the corresponding dose-response curve is non-differentiable at the dose, where the constant, low-dose level (equal to d) abruptly changes into exponential decay. This model is similar to the hockey stick model (Environment Canada, 2005, pp. 108–110; Ritz and Streibig, 2008, p. 41), except that linear decay has been replaced by exponential decay.

B.4.4 Biphasic models with a peak

Recently, two biphasic dose-response models suitable for describing data obtained from biosensors were suggested by Martin-Betancor *et al.* (2015). Like hormesis models, these two models are useful for describing dose-response data showing a non-monotonous behaviour: increasing towards a maximum or peak, where the first phase changes into the second phase, and then decreasing as doses become larger and larger.

The Gaussian model is derived from the density function of the normal distribution:

$$f(x, (b, c, d, e, f)) = c + (d - c)\exp(-\{(x - e)/b\}^f/2)$$

This model may be used to describe biphasic dose-response data that exhibit symmetric behaviour in terms of increase to and decrease from the maximum response level, i.e., same behaviour for both phases.

The log-Gaussian model is defined in a similar way, but due to the logarithmic terms, asymmetry in the behaviour of the two phases (e.g., rapid increase vs. slower decrease) may be incorporated:

$$f(x, (b, c, d, e, f)) = c + (d - c)\exp(-\{|\{\log(x) - \log(e)\}|/b\}^f/2)$$

For both models the parameter f may be useful for capturing varying shapes in the dose-response data.

B.5   Fixing parameters

One key property of *drc* is the hierarchical structure of the built-in model functions, which provides a convenient way to specify special cases obtained by fixing one or more parameters *a priori* at certain given values. These parameters will not be estimated from the data, but will be kept fixed at the specified values. In practice, such special cases occur quite frequently (as seen in Table B.1 and Table B.2).

All built-in model functions in *drc* accept the argument `fixed`, which is used for fixing parameters at given values. For instance, the general five-parameter log-logistic model function may be used for deriving various special cases:

- Fixing $f = 1$:

$$c + \frac{d - c}{1 + \exp(b(\log(x) - \log(e)))}$$

  In *drc*: `LL.5(fixed = c(NA, NA, NA, NA, 1))` or abbreviated `LL.4()`

- Fixing both $f = 1$ and $c = 0$:

$$\frac{d}{1 + \exp(b(\log(x) - \log(e)))}$$

  In *drc*: `LL.4(fixed = c(NA, 0, NA, NA))` or abbreviated `LL.3()`

- Fixing $f = 1$, $c = 0$, and $d = 1$:

$$\frac{1}{1 + \exp(b(\log(x) - \log(e)))}$$

  In *drc*: `LL.4(fixed = c(NA, 0, 1, NA))` or abbreviated `LL.2()`

Note that NAs are used to indicate that parameters are to be estimated from the data. Note also that model parameters come in alphabetical order: b, c, d, e, f, which is assumed when specifying the argument `fixed`.

TABLE B.1
List of more commonly used model functions with the corresponding names in *drc*.

Class	Model name	Number parms	Function in *drc*
Log-logistic			
		4	LL.4()
		3	LL.2()
		2	LL.2()
	Shifted E-max	3	MM.3()
	E-max/Michaelis-Menten	2	MM.2()
	Burr type III	5	LL.5()
Log-normal			
		4	LN.4()
		3	LN.3()
		2	LN.2()
Weibull type 1			
		4	W1.4()
		3	W1.3()
		2	W1.2()
	Exponential decay	3	EXD.3()
		2	EXD.2()
Weibull type 2			
		4	W2.4()
		3	W2.3()
		2	W2.2()
	Asymptotic regression	3	AR.3()
		2	AR.2()
Gamma model		4	gammadr()
Multistage		4	multi2()
NEC			
		4	NEC.4()
		3	NEC.3()
		2	NEC.2()
Biphasic with a peak			
		5	gaussian()
		5	lgaussian()

TABLE B.2
List of more specialized model functions with the corresponding names in *drc*.

Model	Specification	Function in *drc*
Baroflex	Five-parameter	baro5()
Brain-Cousens		
	Five-parameter	BC.5()
	Four-parameter	BC.4()
Cedergreen-Ritz-Streibig	Five-parameter	
	$\alpha = 1$	CRSa.5()
	$\alpha = 0.5$	CRSb.5()
	$\alpha = 0.25$	CRSc.5()
	Four-parameter	
	$\alpha = 1$	CRSa.4()
	$\alpha = 0.5$	CRSb.4()
	$\alpha = 0.25$	CRSc.4()
U-shaped Cedergreen-Ritz-Streibig	Five-parameter	
	$\alpha = 1$	UCRSa.5()
	$\alpha = 0.5$	UCRSb.5()
	$\alpha = 0.25$	UCRSc.5()
	Four-parameter	
	$\alpha = 1$	UCRSa.4()
	$\alpha = 0.5$	UCRSb.4()
	$\alpha = 0.25$	UCRSc.4()
Two-phase model	Seven-parameter	twophase()
Three-phase model	Ten-parameter	threephase()
Fractional polynomial	Four-parameter	
	p_1, p_2	FPL.4()
Universal response surface analysis	Seven-parameter	
		ursa()

Appendix C

R code for plots

In this appendix we provide **R** code for the plotting example where more than a few lines are needed to obtain the result. We use the following extension packages:

```
library(drc)

library(devtools)
install_github("DoseResponse/drcData")
library(drcData)

install_github("DoseResponse/medrc")
library(medrc)

library(ggplot2)
```

C.1   Continuous dose-response data

As dose-response analysis is a type of regression analysis, it is natural to show confidence bands around the fitted regression curve instead of providing error bars at each dose in the dataset.

In this section we provide an example of how functionality of *drc* may be used for constructing a high-quality plot, using the extension package *ggplot2* (Wickham, 2016).

We need a few preparations before being able to do the actual plotting. First we generate dose levels on the logarithmic scale as support for the line using the function expand.grid(). Based on the model fit, the function predict() returns predicted values with confidence intervals for all generated dose levels and everything is gathered in the dataset **newdata**. Finally, plotting doses on a logarithmic scale will result in problems unless we help by shifting the dose 0 slightly upwards.

C.1.1 Ferulic acid as an herbicide

We use *ggplot2* to produce a high-quality plot of the fitted dose-response curve obtained in Subsection 1.1.3.

```
ryegrass.LL.4 <- drm(rootl ~ conc,
                    data = ryegrass,
                    fct = LL.4())


newdata <- expand.grid(conc = exp(seq(log(0.5), log(100),
                                        length = 100)))
pm <- predict(ryegrass.LL.4, newdata = newdata,
            interval = "confidence")
newdata$p <- pm[, 1]
newdata$pmin <- pm[, 2]
newdata$pmax <- pm[, 3]


ryegrass$conc0 <- ryegrass$conc
ryegrass$conc0[ryegrass$conc0 == 0] <- 0.5
```

The functionality of *ggplot2* consists of different building blocks. The plot is initialized with `ggplot()`. Components are added to the initial plot using the + and the different geom functions. We use geoms to add the data points, the predicted curve, and the ribbon presenting the confidence bands. Finally, we specify that the x axis should be rendered on the logarithmic scale (see Figure C.1).

C.2 Estimation of BMD

This section contains **R** lines for some of the plots shown in Chapter 6.

C.2.1 Pathogens in food

The **R** lines used for producing Figure 6.1 in Subsection 6.1.1 are shown below.

```
plot(pathogen.m1,
    broken = TRUE, bp = 10,
    xlab = "Echovirus 12 (pfu)",
    ylab = "Proportion infected",
    xlim = c(0, 100000),
    ylim = c(0, 1),
    axes = FALSE)
```

```
axis(2, c(0.0, 0.1, 0.2, 0.4, 0.6, 0.8, 1),
     c("0.0", "BMR", 0.2, 0.4, 0.6, 0.8, "1.0"))

axis(1,c(90.3, 1000, 10000, 100000),
     c("BMD", "1000", "10000", "100000"))


ggplot(ryegrass, aes(x = conc0, y = rootl)) +
  geom_point() +
  geom_line(data = newdata, aes(x = conc, y=p)) +
  geom_ribbon(data = newdata,
              aes(x = conc, y = p, ymin = pmin, ymax = pmax),
              alpha = 0.2) +
    coord_trans(x = "log") +
  xlab("Ferulic acid (mM)") + ylab("Root length (cm)")
```

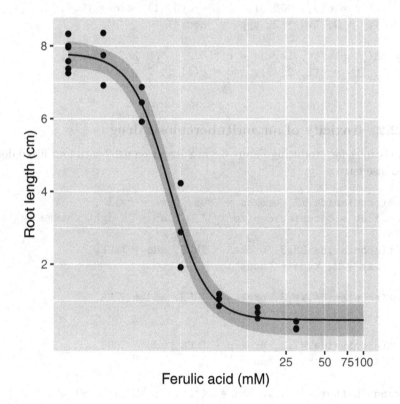

FIGURE C.1
Four-parameter log-logistic model with confidence bands fitted to the dataset
ryegrass.

```
segments(1, 0.1, 90.3, 0.1)

segments(90.3, 0.1, 90.3, -100)
```

Likewise, the **R** lines for showing model averaging in Figure 6.7 in Subsection 6.3.1 look like this:

```
plot(pathogen.m1, broken = TRUE, bp = 10,
    xlab = "Echovirus 12 (pfu)", ylab = "Proportion infected",
    xlim = c(0, 100000), ylim = c(0, 1))

plot(pathogen.LN.2, broken = TRUE, bp = 10,
    xlim = c(0, 100000), ylim = c(0, 1), add = TRUE,
    lty = 2, type = "none")

plot(pathogen.W2.2, broken = TRUE, bp = 10,
    xlim = c(0, 100000), ylim = c(0, 1), add = TRUE,
    lty = 3, lwd = 2, type = "none")

legend("topleft", legend = c("LL.2", "LN.2", "W2.2"),
    lty = c(1, 2, 3), lwd = c(1, 1, 2), bty = "n")
```

C.2.2 Toxicity of an antituberculosis drug

The **R** lines for producing Figure 6.8 in Subsection 6.2.2 with four fitted dose-response curves.

```
plot(aconiazide.m2, broken = TRUE, type = "all",
    xlab = "Aconiazide (mg/kg)", ylab = "Weight change (g)")

plot(aconiazide.LN.3, broken = TRUE, add = TRUE,
    lty = 2, type = "none")

plot(aconiazide.W1.3, broken = TRUE, add = TRUE,
    lty = 3, type = "none")

plot(aconiazide.W2.3, broken = TRUE, add = TRUE,
    lty = 4, type = "none")

legend("bottomleft", legend = c("LL.4", "LN.4", "W1.4", "W2.4"),
    lty = c(1, 2, 3, 4), lwd = c(1, 1, 2, 2), bty = "n")
```

The **R** lines for producing Figure 6.9 in Subsection 6.3.2 are provided below.

```
plot(aconiazide.m2, broken = TRUE, type = "all",
    lty = 2, xlab = "Aconiazide (mg/kg)",
    ylab = "Weight change (g)",
    xlim = c(0, 10000), ylim = c(0, 400))

plot(aconiazide.LN.3, broken = TRUE, add = TRUE,
    lty = 2, type = "none", xlim = c(0, 10000),
    ylim = c(0, 400))

plot(aconiazide.W1.3, broken = TRUE, add = TRUE,
    lty = 2, type = "none", xlim = c(0, 10000),
    ylim = c(0, 400))

plot(aconiazide.W2.3, broken = TRUE, add = TRUE,
    lty = 2, type = "none", xlim = c(0, 10000),
    ylim = c(0, 400))

aconiazide.AIC < -AIC(aconiazide.m2, aconiazide.LN.3,
                aconiazide.W1.3, aconiazide.W2.3)

AICWeights<-exp(-aconiazide.AIC$AIC) /
    sum(exp(-aconiazide.AIC$AIC))

aconiazide.curve <- bmdMACurve(modelList = list(aconiazide.m2,
                    aconiazide.LN.3, aconiazide.W1.3,
                    aconiazide.W2.3),
                    modelWeights = AICWeights, 300)
g <- function(dose){aconiazide.curve$MACurve(dose) + 300}

curve(g, 1, 10000, add = TRUE, lwd = 2)

legend("bottomleft", legend = c("Individual curves",
                    "Model-averaged curve"),
    lty = c(2, 1), lwd = c(1, 2), bty = "n")
```

C.3 Hierarchical nonlinear models

This section contains **R** lines for plots shown in Chapter 7.

C.3.1 Inhibition of photosynthesis in spinach

For the visualization of the predicted dose-response curves in the example with spinach in Section 7.2.2, a dataset with new dose levels for both herbicides needs to be constructed. The *dplyr* and *tidyr* packages provide an infrastructure to modify and tidy data. The pipe operator %>% applies a function on the right-hand side to a dataframe on the left-hand side.

```
library(dplyr)
library(tidyr)
pdata <- spinach %>%
  group_by(CURVE, HERBICIDE) %>%
  expand(DOSE = exp(seq(-5, 5, length = 50)))
```

For each combination of the curve and herbicide indicators, a sequence of 50 new dose levels are created, which are equally spaced on the logarithmic scale. The function `predict()` evaluates the predictions for the new dataframe on the assay level and on the population level for `level=0`.

```
pdata$SLOPEind <- predict(modspinach, newdata = pdata)
pdata$SLOPE <- predict(modspinach, newdata = pdata, level = 0)
```

With the information about each predicted curve in the new dataframe, the package *ggplot2* is used to add the predictions to a scatterplot of the set of observations, shown in Figure 7.2.

```
ggplot(spinach, aes(x = log(DOSE), y = SLOPE,
                    colour = HERBICIDE, group = CURVE,
                    shape = HERBICIDE)) +
  geom_point() +
  geom_line(data = pdata) +
  geom_line(data = pdata, aes(y = SLOPEind), linetype = 2) +
  theme_bw() +
  scale_colour_grey(start = 0.1, end = 0.6) +
  scale_x_continuous("DOSE",
                    breaks = log(c(0.01, 0.1, 1, 10, 100)),
                    labels = c(0.01, 0.1, 1, 10, 100))
```

C.3.2 Herbicides with auxin effects

For the visualization of the predicted curves of the Auxins example in Section 7.2.3, a new dataset is constructed with new dose levels at each combination of the dummy-coded grouping, which is created in the user-defined design matrix. The common control level is excluded from the new dataset. The package *ggplot2* is used to draw a scatterplot in Figure 7.2, adding lines for the predictions on the individual replicate and population level.

```
library(dplyr)
library(tidyr)
pauxdata <- auxins %>%
  group_by(replicate, herbicide, formulation,
           h24D, mp, dp, comm, h24Dcomm, mpcomm, dpcomm) %>%
  expand(dose=exp(seq(-4, 0, length = 25)))
pauxdata <- subset(pauxdata, formulation != "control")

pauxdata$yind <- predict(auxmod, newdata = pauxdata)
pauxdata$y <- predict(auxmod, newdata = pauxdata, level = 0)

ggplot(subset(auxins, formulation != "control"),
       aes(y = dryweight, x = log(dose),
           colour = herbicide, shape = herbicide)) +
  geom_point() +
  geom_line(data = pauxdata, aes(y = y)) +
  geom_line(data = pauxdata, aes(y = yind,
                                 group = replicate:herbicide),
            lty = 2) +
  facet_wrap(~ formulation) +
  theme_bw() +
  scale_colour_grey(start = 0.8, end = 0.2) +
  scale_x_continuous("dose",
                     breaks = log(c(0.02, 0.05, 0.15, 0.4, 1)),
                     labels = c(0.02, 0.05, 0.15, 0.4, 1))
```

C.3.3 Drought stress resistance in *Brassica oleracea*

The following **R** code is used to construct the scatterplot in Figure 7.3 in Section 7.2.4.

```
library(dplyr)
library(tidyr)
pbroc <- broccoli %>%
  group_by(Stress, Genotype, ID) %>%
  expand(Day = seq(1, 16, length = 25))
pbroc$ygeno <- predict(brmod, newdata = pbroc)

ggplot(broccoli,
       aes(y = LeafLength, x = Day,
           linetype = Stress, group = ID)) +
  geom_line(colour = "grey") +
  geom_line(data = pbroc, aes(y = ygeno)) +
  facet_wrap(~ Genotype) +
  theme_bw()
```

Bibliography

Aranda-Ordaz, F. J. (1981). On two families of transformation to additivity for binary response. *Biometrika* **68**, 357–363.

Bailer, A. J., Noble, R. B. and Wheeler, M. W. (2005). Model uncertainty and risk estimation for experimental studies of quantal responses. *Risk Analysis* **25**, 291–299.

Bailer, A. J. and Oris, J. T. (1997). Estimating inhibition concentrations for different response scales using generalized linear models. *Environmental Toxicology and Chemistry* **16**, 1554–1559.

Beckon, W. N., Parkins, C., Maximovich, A. and Beckon, A. V. (2008). A general approach to modeling biphasic relationships. *Environmental Science & Technology* **42**, 1308–1314.

Begg, C. B. and Gray, R. (1984). Calculation of polychotomous logistic regression parameters using individualized regressions. *Biometrika* **71**, 11–18.

Beland, F. A., Dooley, K. L., Hansen, E. B. and Sheldon, W. G. (1995). Six-month toxicity comparison of the antituberculosis drugs aconiazide and isoniazid in Fischer 344 rats. *Journal of the American College of Toxicology* **14**, 328–342.

Belz, R. G. and Piepho, H.-P. (2012). Modeling effective dosages in hormetic dose-response studies. *PLoS ONE* **10**, e33432.

Bentley, K. S., Kirkland, D., Murphy, M. and Marshall, R. (2000). Evaluation of thresholds for benomyl- and carbendazim-induced aneuploidy in cultured human lymphocytes using fluorescence in situ hybridization. *Mutation Research/Genetic Toxicology and Environmental Mutagenesis* **464**, 41–51.

Berkey, C. S., Hoaglin, D. C., Antczak-Bouckoms, A., Mosteller, F. and Colditz, G. A. (1998). Meta-analysis of multiple outcomes by regression with random effects. *Statistics in Medicine* **17**, 2537–2550.

Brain, P. and Cousens, R. (1989). An equation to describe dose responses where there is stimulation of growth at low dose. *Weed Research* **29**, 93–96.

Bruce, R. D. and Versteeg, D. J. (1992). A statistical procedure for modeling continuous toxicity data. *Environmental Toxicology and Chemistry* **11**, 1485–1494.

Buckland, S. T., Burnham, K. P. and Augustin, N. H. (1997). Model selection: An integral part of inference. *Biometrics* **53**, 603–618.

Buckley, B. E., Piegorsch, W. W. and West, R. W. (2009). Confidence limits on one-stage model parameters in benchmark risk assessment. *Environmental and Ecological Statistics* **16**, 53–62.

Budtz-Jørgensen, E., Keiding, N. and Grandjean, P. (2001). Benchmark dose calculation from epidemiological data. *Biometrics* **57**, 698–706.

Cabanne, F., Gaudry, J. and Streibig, J. (1999). Influence of alkyl oleates on efficacy of phenmedipham applied as an acetone: Water solution on *Galium aparine*. *Weed Research* **39**, 57–67.

Carroll, R. J. and Ruppert, D. (1984). Power transformations when fitting theoretical models to data. *Journal of the American Statistical Association* **79**, 321–328.

Carroll, R. J. and Ruppert, D. (1988). *Transformations and Weighting in Regression*. Chapman & Hall, London, first edn.

Caux, P.-Y. and Moore, D. R. (1997). A spreadsheet program for estimating low toxic effects. *Environmental Toxicology and Chemistry* **16**, 802–806.

Cedergreen, N., Ritz, C. and Streibig, J. C. (2005). Improved empirical models describing hormesis. *Environmental Toxicology and Chemistry* **24**, 3166–3172.

Chapman, G. A., Denton, D. L. and Lazorchak, J. M. (1995). *Short-Term Methods for Estimating the Chronic Toxicity of Effluents and Receiving Waters to West Coast Marine and Estuarine Organisms*. U. S. EPA.

Christensen, M. G., Teicher, H. B. and Streibig, J. C. (2003). Linking fluorescence induction curve and biomass in herbicide screening. *Pest Management Science* **59**, 1303–1310.

Cornou, C., Storm, I. M. D., Hindrichsen, I. K., Worgan, H., Bakewell, E., Ruiz, D. R. Y., Abecia, L., Tagliapietra, F., Cattani, M., Ritz, C. *et al.* (2013). A ring test of a wireless in vitro gas production system. *Animal Production Science* **53**, 585–592.

Crump, K. S. (1984). A new method for determining allowable daily intakes. *Fundamental and Applied Toxicology* **4**, 854–871.

Davidian, M. and Giltinan, D. M. (1995). *Nonlinear Models for Repeated Measurement Data*. Chapman & Hall, Boca Raton, Florida.

Davison, A. C. and Hinkley, D. V. (1997). *Bootstrap Methods and Their Application*. Cambridge University Press, Cambridge.

Delignette-Muller, M. L., Lopes, C., Veber, P. and Charles, S. (2014a). Calculation of polychotomous logistic regression parameters using individualized regressions. *Environmental Science & Technology* **48**, 7544–7551.

Delignette-Muller, M. L., Lopes, C., Veber, P. and Charles, S. (2014b). Statistical handling of reproduction data for exposure-response modeling. *Environmetal Science & Technology* **48**, 7544–7551.

Demidenko, E. (2013). *Mixed Models: Theory and Applications with R*. Wiley Series in Probability and Statistics. John Wiley & Sons, Inc., Hoboken, NJ, USA, 2nd edn.

DiCiccio, T. J. and Efron, B. (1996). Bootstrap confidence intervals (with discussion). *Statistical Science* **11**, 189–228.

Downs, T. (1992). Biostatistical approaches for modeling U-shaped dose-response curves and study design considerations in assessing the biological effects of low doses. In *Biological Effects of Low Level Exposures to Chemicals and Radiation* (ed. E. J. Calabrese), 119–145. Lewis Publishers, Boca Raton, Florida. Chapter 7.

Edler, L. and Kopp-Schneider, A. (1998). Statistical models for low dose exposure. *Mutation Research* **405**, 227–236.

Environment Canada (2005). *Guidance Document on Statistical Methods for Environmental Toxicity Tests*. Environment Canada, Ottawa.

van Ewijk, P. H. and Hoekstra, J. A. (1993). Calculation of the EC50 and its confidence interval when subtoxic stimulus is present. *Ecotoxicology and Environmental Safety* **25**, 25–32.

Faes, C., Aerts, M., Geys, H. and Molenberghs, G. (2007). Model averaging using fractional polynomials to estimate a safe level of exposure. *Risk Analysis* **27**, 111–123.

Fang, C. and Zhang, D. (2014). Estimating the interaction index in drug combination experiments. *Statistics in Biopharmaceutical Research* **6**, 144–153.

Fang, Q., Piegorsch, W. W. and Barnes, K. Y. (2015). Bayesian benchmark dose analysis. *Environmetrics* **26**, 373–382.

Faraggi, D., Izikson, P. and Reiser, B. (2003). Confidence intervals for the 50 per cent response dose. *Statistics in Medicine* **22**, 1977–1988.

Feng, Z. and McCulloch, C. E. (1992). Statistical inference using maximum likelihood estimation and the generalized likelihood ratio when the true parameter is on the boundary of the parameter space. *Statistics & Probability Letters* **13**, 325–332.

Finney, D. J. (1949). The estimation of the parameters of tolerance distributions. *Biometrika* **36**, 239–256.

Finney, D. J. (1971). *Probit Analysis*. Cambridge University Press, London, third edn.

Finney, D. J. (1979). Bioassay and the practice of statistical inference. *International Statistical Review* **47**, 1–12.

Fox, D. R. and Landis, W. G. (2016). Don't be fooled - a no-observed-effect concentration is no substitute for a poor concentration-response experiment. *Environmental Toxicology and Chemistry* **35**, 2141–2148.

Fox, J. F., Hogan, K. A. and Davis, A. (2017). Dose-response modeling with summary data from developmental toxicity studies. *Risk Analysis* **37**, 905–917.

Garnier-Laplace, J., Della-Vedova, C., Andersson, P., Copplestone, D., Cailes, C., Beresford, N. A., Howard, B. J., Howe, P. and Whitehouse, P. (2010). A multi-criteria weight of evidence approach for deriving ecological benchmarks for radioactive substances. *Journal of Radiological Protection* **30**, 215.

Gaylor, D. W. and Slikker, W. (1990). Risk assessment for neurotoxic effects. *Neurotoxicology* **11**, 211–8.

Gong, X., Zeng, R., Luo, S., Yong, C. and Zheng, Q. (2004). Two new secalonic acids from *Aspergillus Japonicus* and their allelopathic effects on higher plants. In *Proceedings of International Symposium on Allelopathy Research and Application, 27-29 April, Shanshui, Guangdong, China* (eds. R. Zeng and S. Luo), 209–217.

Gottschalk, P. G. and Dunn, J. R. (2005). The five-parameter logistic: A characterization and comparison with the four-parameter logistic. *Analytical Biochemistry* **343**, 54–65.

Hardy, A., Benford, D., Halldorsson, T., Jeger, M. J., Knutsen, K. H., More, S., Mortensen, A., Naegeli, H., Noteborn, H., Ockleford, C., Ricci, A., Rychen, G., Silano, V., Solecki, R., Turck, D., Aerts, M., Bodin, L., Davis, A., Edler, L., Gundert-Remy, U., Sand, S., Slob, W., Bottex, B., Abrahantes, J. C., Marques, D. C., Kass, G. and Schlatter, J. R. (2017). Update: Use of the benchmark dose approach in risk assessment. *EFSA Journal* **15**, 4658.

Hesterberg, T. C. (2015). What teachers should know about the bootstrap: Resampling in the undergraduate statistics curriculum. *The American Statistician* **69**, 371–386.

Hoekstra, J. A. (1987). Acute bioassays with control natural mortality. *Water, Air, and Soil Pollution* **35**, 311–317.

van der Hoeven, N. (1997). How to measure no effect. Part III: Statistical aspects of NOEC, ECx and NEC estimates. *Environmetrics* **8**, 255–261.

Hothorn, T., Bretz, F. and Westfall, P. (2008). Simultaneous inference in general parametric models. *Biometrical Journal* **50**, 346–363.

van Houwelingen, H. C., Arends, L. R. and Stijnen, T. (2002). Advanced methods in meta-analysis: Multivariate approach and meta-regression. *Statistics in Medicine* **21**, 589–624.

Huber, P. J. (1981). *Robust Statistics*. John Wiley & Sons, Hoboken.

Inderjit, Streibig, J. C. and Olofsdotter, M. (2002). Joint action of phenolic acid mixtures and its significance in allelopathy research. *Physiologia Plantarum* **114**, 422–428.

Izadi, H., Grundy, J. E. and Bose, R. (2012). Evaluation of the Benchmark Dose for Point of Departure Determination for a Variety of Chemical Classes in Applied Regulatory Settings. *Risk Analysis* **32**, 830–835.

Jager, T., Albert, C., Preuss, T. G. and Ashauer, R. (2011). General unified threshold model of Survival – a toxicokinetic-toxicodynamic framework for ecotoxicology. *Environmental Science & Technology* **45**, 2529–2540.

Jensen, S. M., Andreasen, C., Streibig, J. C., Keshtkar, E. and Ritz, C. (2017). A note on the analysis of germination data from complex experimental designs. *Seed Science Research* **27**, 321–327.

Jensen, S. M. and Ritz, C. (2015). Simultaneous inference for model averaging of derived parameters. *Risk Analysis* **35**, 68–76.

Jensen, S. M. and Ritz, C. (2018). A comparison of approaches for simultaneous inference of fixed effects for multiple outcomes using linear mixed models. *Statistics in Medicine* **37**, 2474–2486.

Jeske, D. R., Xu, H. K., Blessinger, T., Jensen, P. and Trumble, J. (2009). Testing for the equality of EC50 values in the presence of unequal slopes with application to toxicity of selenium types. *Journal of Agricultural, Biological, and Environmental Statistics* **14**, 469–483.

Jiang, X. and Kopp-Schneider, A. (2014). Summarizing EC50 estimates from multiple dose-response experiments: A comparison of a meta-analysis strategy to a mixed-effects model approach. *Biometrical Journal* **56**, 493–512.

Kalaian, H. A. and Raudenbush, S. W. (1996). A multivariate mixed linear model for meta-analysis. *Psychological Methods* **1**, 227–235.

Kang, S.-H., Kodell, R. L. and Chen, J. J. (2000). Incorporating model uncertainties along with data uncertainties in microbial risk assessment. *Regulatory Toxicology and Pharmacology* **32**, 68–72.

Keller, F., Giehl, M., Czock, D. and Zellner, D. (2002). PK-PD curve-fitting problems with the Hill equation? Try one of the 1-exp functions derived from Hodgkin, Douglas or Gompertz. *International Journal of Clinical Pharmacology and Therapeutics* **40**, 23–29.

Kerr, D. R. and Meador, J. P. (1996). Modeling dose response using generalized linear models. *Environmental Toxicology and Chemistry* **15**, 395–401.

Keshtkar, E., Mathiassen, S. K., Beffa, R. and Kudsk, P. (2017). Seed germination and seedling emergence of blackgrass (*Alopecurus myosuroides*) as affected by non–target-site herbicide resistance. *Weed Science* **65**, 732–742.

Kociba, R., Keyes, D., Beyer, J., Carreon, R., Wade, C., Dittenber, D., Kalnins, R., Frauson, L., Park, C., Barnard, S., Hummel, R. and Humiston, C. (1978). Results of a two-year chronic toxicity and oncogenicity study of 2,3,7,8-tetrachlorodibenzo-p-dioxin in rats. *Toxicology and Applied Pharmacology* **46**, 279–303.

Kodell, R. L. and West, R. W. (1993). Upper confidence limits on excess risk for quantitative responses. *Risk Analysis* **13**, 177–182.

Kooijman, S. (1981). Parametric analyses of mortality rates in bioassays. *Water Research* **15**, 107–119.

Kratzer, D. D. and Littell, R. C. (2004). Appropriate statistical methods to compare dose responses of methionine sources. *Poultry Science* **85**, 947–954.

Lindstrom, M. J. and Bates, D. M. (1990). Nonlinear mixed effects models for repeated measures data. *Biometrics* **46**, 673.

MacDougall, J. (2006). Analysis of dose–response Studies – Emax model. In *Dose Finding in Drug Development* (ed. N. Ting). Springer.

Martin-Betancor, K., Ritz, C., Fernández-Piñas, F., Leganés, F. and Rodea-Palomares, I. (2015). Defining an additivity framework for mixture research in inducible whole-cell biosensors. *Scientific Reports* **5**, 17200.

McCullagh, P. and Nelder, J. A. (1989). *Generalized Linear Models*. Chapman & Hall, Boca Raton, Florida, second edn.

Meister, R. and van den Brink, P. J. (2000). The analysis of laboratory toxicity experiments (Chapter 4). In *Statistics in Ecotoxicology* (ed. T. Sparks), 99–118. John Wiley & Sons, Chichester.

Meister, R. and den Brink, P. J. V. (2000). The analysis of laboratory toxicity experiments. In *Statistics in Ecotoxicology* (ed. T. Sparks), 99–118. Wiley.

Moon, H., Kim, S. B., Chen, J. J., George, N. I. and Kodell, R. L. (2013). Model uncertainty and model averaging in the estimation of infectious doses for microbial pathogens. *Risk Analysis* **33**, 220–231.

Morgan, B. J. T. (1992). *Analysis of Quantal Response Data*. Chapman & Hall.

Morgan, B. J. T. and Smith, D. M. (1992). A note on Wadley's problem with overdispersion. *Applied Statistics* **41**, 349–354.

Murrell, J. A., Portier, C. J. and Morris, R. W. (1998). Characterizing dose-response i: Critical assessment of the benchmark dose concept. *Risk Analysis* **18**, 13–26.

Namata, H., Aerts, M., Faes, C. and Teunis, P. (2008). Model averaging in microbial risk assessment using fractional polynomials. *Risk Analysis* **28**, 891–905.

Nash, J. C. (2014). On best practice optimization methods in R. *Journal of Statistical Software* **60**, 1–14.

National Toxicology Program (2006). NTP technical report on the toxicology and carcinogenesis studies of 2,3,7,8-tetrachlorodibenzo-p-dioxin (TCDD) (CAS No. 1746-01-6) in female Harlan Sprague-Dawley rats (Gavage Studies). *National Toxicology Program Technical Report Series* 4–232.

Nellemann, C., Majken, D., Lam, H. R. and Vinggaard, A. M. (2003). The combined effects of vinclozolin and procymidone do not deviate from expected additivity in vitro and in vivo. *Toxicological Sciences* **71**, 251–262.

Normolle, D. (1993). An algorithm for robust non-linear analysis of radioimmunoassays and other bioassays. *Statistics in Medicine* **12**, 2025–2042.

Nottingham, Q. J. and Birch, J. B. (2000). A semiparametric approach to analysing dose-response data. *Statistics in Medicine* **19**, 389–404.

OECD (2006). *Current Approaches in the Statistical Analysis of Ecotoxicity Data: A Guidance to application - Annexes*. Organisation for Economic Co-operation and Development. OECD Environment Health and Safety Publications, Series on Testing and Assessment, No. 54.

Pant, M. D. and Headrick, T. C. (2013). A method for simulating Burr Type III and Type XII distributions through *l*-moments and *l*-correlations. *ISRN Applied Mathematics* Article ID 191604.

Piegorsch, W. W. and Bailer, A. J. (2005). *Analyzing Environmental Data*. John Wiley & Sons, Chichester.

Piegorsch, W. W., Xiong, H., Bhattacharya, R. N. and Lin, L. (2012). Nonparametric estimation of benchmark doses in environmental risk assessment. *Environmetrics* **23**, 717–728.

Piegorsch, W. W., Xiong, H., Bhattacharya, R. N. and Lin, L. (2014). Benchmark dose analysis via nonparametric regression modeling. *Risk Analysis* **34**, 135–151.

Pinheiro, J. C. and Bates, D. M. (2000). *Mixed-Effects Models in S and S-PLUS*. Statistics and Computing. Springer-Verlag, New York.

Pipper, C. B., Ritz, C. and Bisgaard, H. (2012). A versatile method for confirmatory evaluation of the effects of a covariate in multiple models. *Applied Statistics* **61**, 315–326.

Pires, A. M., Branco, J. A., Picado, A. and Mendonça, E. (2002). Models for the estimation of a "no effect concentration." *Environmetrics* **13**, 15–27.

Prentice, R. L. (1976). A generalization of the probit and logit methods for dose response curves. *Biometrics* **32**, 761–768.

R Core Team (2018). *R: A Language and Environment for Statistical Computing*. R Foundation for Statistical Computing, Vienna, Austria.

Racine, A., Grieve, A. P., Fluhler, H. and Smith, A. F. M. (1986). Bayesian methods in practice: Experiences in the pharmaceutical industry. *Applied Statistics* **35**, 93–150.

Racine-Poon, A. (1988). A Bayesian approach to nonlinear calibration problems. *Journal of the American Statistical Association* **83**, 650–656.

Ricketts, J. H. and Head, G. A. (1999). A five-parameter logistic equation for investigating asymmetry of curvature in baroreflex studies. *American Journal of Physiology (Regulatory Integrative Comp. Physiol. 46)* **277**, 441–454.

Ringblom, J., Johanson, G. and Öberg, M. (2014). Current modeling practice may lead to falsely high benchmark dose estimates. *Regulatory Toxicology and Pharmacology* **69**, 171–177.

Ritz, C. (2010). Towards a unified approach to dose-response modeling in ecotoxicology. *Environmental Toxicology and Chemistry* **29**, 220–229.

Ritz, C., Baty, F., Streibig, J. C. and Gerhard, D. (2015). Dose-response analysis using R. *PLoS ONE* **10**, e0146021.

Ritz, C., Cedergreen, N., Jensen, J. E. and Streibig, J. C. (2006). Relative potency in nonsimilar dose-response curves. *Weed Science* **54**, 407–412.

Ritz, C., Gerhard, D. and Hothorn, L. A. (2013a). A unified framework for benchmark dose estimation applied to mixed models and model averaging. *Statistics in Biopharmaceutical Research* **5**, 79–90.

Ritz, C., Pipper, C. B. and Streibig, J. C. (2013b). Analysis of germination data from agricultural experiments. *European Journal of Agronomy* **45**, 1–6.

Ritz, C. and Streibig, J. C. (2005). Bioassay analysis using R. *Journal of Statistical Software* **12**, 1–22.

Ritz, C. and Streibig, J. C. (2008). *Nonlinear Regression with R.* useR! series. Springer, New York.

Ritz, C. and Van der Vliet, L. (2009). Handling non-normality and variance heterogeneity for quantitative sublethal toxicity tests. *Environmental Toxicology and Chemistry* **28**, 2009–2017.

Royston, P. and Altman, D. G. (1994). Regression using fractional polynomials of continuous covariates: Parsimonious parametric modelling. *Applied Statistics* **43**, 429–467.

Sand, S., Filipsson, A. F. and Victorin, K. (2002). Evaluation of the benchmark dose method for dichotomous data: Model dependence and model selection. *Regulatory Toxicology and Pharmacology* **36**, 184–197.

Sand, S., von Rosen, D., Victorin, K. and Filipsson, A. F. (2006). Identification of a critical dose level for risk assessment: Developments in benchmark dose analysis of continuous endpoints. *Toxicological Sciences* **90**, 241–251.

Sand, S., Victorin, K. and Filipsson, A. F. (2008). The current state of knowledge on the use of the benchmark dose concept in risk assessment. *Journal of Applied Toxicology* **28**, 405–421.

Scholze, M., Boedeker, W., Faust, M., Backhaus, T., Altenburger, R. and Grimme, L. H. (2001). A general best-fit method for concentration-response curves and the estimation of low-effect concentrations. *Environmental Toxicology and Chemistry* **20**, 448–457.

Seber, G. A. F. and Wild, C. J. (1989). *Nonlinear Regression.* John Wiley & Sons, New York.

Shao, K. (2012). A comparison of three methods for integrating historical information for Bayesian model averaged benchmark dose estimation. *Environmental Toxicology and Pharmacology* **34**, 288–296.

Shao, Q. (2000). Estimation for hazardous concentrations based on NOEC toxicity data: An alternative approach. *Environmetrics* **11**, 583–595.

Slob, W. (2002). Dose-response modeling of continuous endpoints. *Toxicological Sciences* **66**, 298–312.

Stephenson, G. L., Koper, N., Atkinson, G. F., Solomon, K. R. and Scroggins, R. P. (2000). Use of nonlinear regression techniques for describing concentration-response relationships of plant species exposed to contaminated site soils. *Environmental Toxicology and Chemistry* **19**, 2968–2981.

Streibig, J. C. (1981). A method for determining the biological effect of herbicide mixtures. *Weed Science* **29**, 469–473.

Streibig, J. C. (1983). Joint action of root-absorbed mixtures of dpx-4189 and linuron in *Sinapis alba* l. and barley. *Weed Research* **23**, 3–9.

Streibig, J. C. (1987). Joint action of root-absorbed mixtures of auxin herbicides in *Sinapis alba* L. and barley (*Hordeum vulgare* L.). *Weed Research* **27**, 337–347.

Streibig, J. C., Dayan, F. E., Rimando, A. M. and Duke, S. O. (1999). Joint action of natural and synthetic photosystem II inhibitors. *Pesticide Science* **55**, 137–146.

Streibig, J. C. and Jensen, J. E. (2000). Actions of herbicides in mixtures. In *Herbicides and Their Mechanisms of Action*. Sheffield Academic Press, Sheffield.

Streibig, J. C., Rudemo, M. and Jensen, J. E. (1993). Dose-response curves and statistical models. In *Herbicide Bioassays* (eds. J. C. Streibig and P. Kudsk), 29–55. CRC Press, Boca Raton.

Strodl Andersen, J., Holst, H., Spliid, H., Andersen, H., Baun, A. and Nyholm, N. (1998). Continuous ecotoxicological data evaluated relative to a control response. *Journal of Agricultural, Biological, and Environmental Statistics* **3**, 405–420.

Stromberg, A. J. (1993). Computation of high breakdown nonlinear regression parameters. *Journal of the American Statistical Association* **88**, 237–244.

Stukel, T. A. (1988). Generalized logistic models. *Journal of the American Statistical Association* **83**, 426–431.

Szöcs, E. and Schäfer, R. B. (2015). Ecotoxicology is not normal. *Environmental Science and Pollution Research* **22**, 13990–13999.

Trajstman, A. C. (1989). Indices for comparing decontaminants when data come from dose-response survival and contamination experiments. *Applied Statistics* **38**, 481–494.

U. S. EPA (2012). *Benchmark Dose Technical Guidance*. 1–99.

Uptmoor, R., Osei-Kwarteng, M., Guertler, S. and Stuetzel, H. (2009). Modeling the effects of drought stress on leaf development in a *Brassica oleracea* doubled haploid population using two-phase linear functions. *Journal of the American Society for Horticultural Sciences* **134**, 543–552.

van der Vaart, A. W. (1998). *Asymptotic Statistics*. Cambridge University Press, Cambridge.

Van der Vliet, L. and Ritz, C. (2013). Statistics for analyzing ecotoxicity test data. In *Encyclopedia of Aquatic Ecotoxicology* (eds. J. Férard and C. Blaise), 1081–1096. Springer, New York.

Venables, W. N. and Ripley, B. D. (2002). *Modern Applied Statistics with S.* Springer, New York, fourth edn. ISBN 0-387-95457-0.

Viechtbauer, W. (2010). Conducting Meta-Analyses in R with the metafor Package. *Journal of Statistical Software* **36**, 1–48.

Vindimian, E., Robaut, C. and Fillion, G. (1983). A method for cooperative or noncooperative binding studies using nonlinear regression analysis on a microcomputer. *Journal of Applied Biochemistry* **5**, 261–268.

Vølund, A. (1978). Application of the four-parameter logistic model to bioassay: Comparison with slope ratio and parallel line models. *Biometrics* **34**, 357–365.

Weisberg, S. (2005). *Applied Linear Regression.* John Wiley & Sons, New York, third edn.

West, R. W., Piegorsch, W. W., Peña, E. A., An, L., Wu, W., Wickens, A. A., Xiong, H. and Chen, W. (2012). The impact of model uncertainty on benchmark dose estimation. *Environmetrics* **23**, 706–716.

Wheeler, M. W. and Bailer, A. J. (2007). Properties of model-averaged BMDLs: A study of model averaging in dichotomous response risk estimation. *Risk Analysis* **27**, 659–670.

Wheeler, M. W. and Bailer, A. J. (2009). Comparing model averaging with other model selection strategies for benchmark dose estimation. *Environmental and Ecological Statistics* **16**, 37–51.

Wheeler, M. W., Bailer, A. J. *et al.* (2008). Model averaging software for dichotomous dose response risk estimation. *Journal of Statistical Software* **26**, 1–15.

Wheeler, M. W., Park, R. M. and Bailer, A. J. (2006). Comparing median lethal concentration values using confidence interval overlap or ratio tests. *Environmental Toxicology and Chemistry* **25**, 1441–1444.

White, H. (1981). Consequences and detection of misspecified nonlinear regression models. *Journal of the American Statistical Association* **76**, 419–433.

White, H. (1996). *Estimation, Inference and Specification Analysis.* Cambridge University Press, Cambridge.

WHO (2005). *The WHO Recommended Classification of Pesticides by Hazard and Guidelines to Classification 2004.* World Health Organisation, Geneva.

Wickham, H. (2016). *ggplot2: Elegant Graphics for Data Analysis.* Springer-Verlag New York. URL http://ggplot2.org.

Yu, Z.-F. and Catalano, P. J. (2005). Quantitative risk assessment for multivariate continuous outcomes with application to neurotoxicology: The bi-
variate case. *Biometrics* **61**, 757–766.

Zeileis, A. (2006). Object-oriented computation of sandwich estimators. *Journal of Statistical Software* **16**, 1–16.

Zeileis, A. and Hothorn, T. (2002). Diagnostic checking in regression relationships. *R News* **2**, 7–10.

Zhu, Y., Wang, T. and Jelsovsky, J. Z. (2007). Bootstrap estimation of benchmark doses and confidence limits with clustered quantal data. *Risk Analysis*
27, 447–465.

Index

Printed in the United States
by Baker & Taylor Publisher Services